What readers say

*Marvelous and long overdue! I am honored to endorse **Beyond Erections**. I think it should be required reading for everyone who is diagnosed with prostate cancer.*

Dr Lorraine Becker (MD), Family Doctor
Fellow of European Committee of Sexual Medicine

☀

*This book is a key read for any man finding erections difficult or even impossible. In addition, I would highly recommend **Beyond Erections** to any person who supports patients with their sexual function, not only to gain an insight into the struggles people face but also so that they can learn how to support them along their new journey.*

Stuart Dawe-Long (FIBMS, MSc, PGCert, BSc)
Senior Clinical Andrologist (Registered Clinical Scientist)
Diplomate of the Institute of Psychosexual Medicine

☀

A profoundly impactful and refreshing exploration of sexual intimacy, challenging the conventional norms that often marginalize those experiencing erectile differences. Mish empowers readers to explore alternative forms of intimate pleasure. His practical tips and inclusive perspective make him a true sexual pleasure warrior.

Delene van Dyk, Professional Registered Nurse
Psychosexual Educator and Counsellor

Well illustrated and easy to understand advice, suggestions, and practices make the journey through this book both pleasurable and comforting.

*Having a guide like this, **Beyond Erections** will open the door to your sexual rejuvenation.*

Steve Jones
Author- Words woke me- my prostate cancer journey in poetry

☀

The book feels like a supportive chat with someone who genuinely gets it. It's encouraging, non-judgmental, and totally normalises what can feel like an awkward topic.

***Beyond Erections** is an honest, empowering, and inclusive guide for anyone navigating erectile differences. Mish Middelmann combines personal experience with practical strategies to create a compassionate and transformative resource. This book is a must-read for men and their partners seeking to redefine intimacy and embrace new possibilities for connection and pleasure.*

Martin Wells, community activist, educator and co-founder of
Out with Prostate Cancer

Beyond Erections

*Sexual pleasure and intimacy
with erectile differences*

by Mish Middelmann

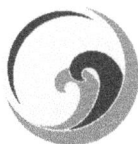

Waves Press

Beyond Erections
Copyright © 2025 by Mish Middelmann
Waves Press, Toronto, Canada
www.beyonderections.com

Paperback ISBN:	978-1-0692760-2-5
Kindle eBook ISBN:	978-1-0692760-3-2
Kobo eBook ISBN:	978-1-0692760-4-9

Cover art: Nudes by Beth www.nudesbybeth.myportfolio.com

Illustrations by Lakshmi S artsyls.studio@gmail.com

Release 1.10

Dedication

To my beloved Colleen, fellow adventurer through this tumultuous life.

For men subtly diminished by non-conforming bodies.

Contents

Foreword 1

Chapter 1 Introduction 3

   1.1   Medical considerations 4
   1.2   Relationship challenges 4
   1.3   Recalibrating sexual signals 6
   1.4   Getting practical 6
   1.5   Language and sources 7
   1.6   Accepting changes in shape 8
   1.7   Personal stories that connect us 9
   1.8   Men are opening up 11
   1.9   Further exploration 12

Chapter 2 Mindset 15

   2.1   Good sex doesn't require a hard penis 15
   2.2   Unshaming erectile difference 17
   2.3   Different strokes for different folks 18
   2.4   What has been lost 20
   2.5   Let go of comparison 21
   2.6   Compassionate invitation 22
   2.7   Sex dates 22
   2.8   Shifting energies and eagerness 23
   2.9   Further exploration 24

Chapter 3 Pleasure 27

   3.1   Preparing to enjoy a soft penis 28
   3.2   Taking touch further 30
   3.3   Penetrating with a soft penis 41
   3.4   Expanding your erotic landscape 44
   3.5   Toys, medicines and other non-human helpers ...54
   3.6   Further exploration 62

Chapter 4 Satisfaction 65

   4.1   Erotic imagination 66
   4.2   Energy circuits fuel sensual lovemaking 68
   4.3   Having hot sex with a soft penis 71

4.4	Evolving orgasms	73
4.5	Redefining orgasm	77
4.6	Holistic satisfaction	79
4.7	Further exploration	79

Chapter 5 We are not alone ... **81**

5.1	Speak out about your experience	81
5.2	Inform yourself	82
5.3	Get help for your relationship	83
5.4	Find people who can help you	84
5.5	Supportive communities	85
5.6	Tracking progress	85
5.7	Further exploration	86

Chapter 6 Action ... **89**

Chapter 7 Resources ... **91**

7.1	Free online resources	91
7.2	Online resources you might consider paying for	92
7.3	Sex aids	92
7.4	Support groups with free membership	93
7.5	Professional helpers	93
7.6	More about quotes in the book	94
7.7	Bibliography	94

Acknowledgements ... **103**

About the author ... **105**

Foreword

I've been Mish's intimate partner since 1982, from the heady days of the hot, lustful sex of a new relationship, through the excitements, complexities, and rewards of having two children together, and now the richness and challenges of navigating sex with aging and erectile differences following his prostatectomy and time.

Mish approached the diagnosis of prostate cancer, surgery, and recovery with his exceptional energy and positivity. Within weeks of diagnosis, he was searching the internet and exploring information about recovery of all bodily functions wherever he could find it – leading him to talk to medical practitioners and other prostate cancer survivors around the world.

Beyond Erections comes from his and our experiences with sex without his penis being hard. Having journalled regularly through much of his life, he has fully documented his journey of discovery. He turned his journal entries into blog posts on his RecoveringMan.net website. Through discussions with many men through Recovering Man support groups, he and others have shared and compared experiences. Mish found that many men had no idea how to move into a different form of sexual expression and experience than they had been used to, and that they and their partners were often suffering through the trauma.

Being unfailingly proactive, Mish wants to try almost anything that has been suggested as an alternative way of being actively sexual with his new body. It's important to both of us that our relationship continues to develop in healthy, happy ways sexually and otherwise, so he's been open and shared his newfound knowledge, ideas, and devices. We've tried much together, and both of us have expanded our awareness of what makes us feel good, what leaves us indifferent, and where we come up against a hard no (this usually comes sooner for me than for Mish!). But whatever we try, we continue to communicate, and this keeps our relationship in good shape.

From my experience, I strongly encourage those with soft penises for any reason to talk openly with their partners, and for partners of those with soft penises to start discovering how to have a satisfying sex life. He has provided suggestions for both physical and more esoteric activities to help you become more conscious of yourself as a sexual being in your current situation. As Mish says in the book, treat it as a buffet – try anything that looks appealing, and leave what doesn't. Come back for more when you're ready.

I'm excited that our experiences may be useful to others!

Colleen Dawson
Toronto, Canada
January 2025

Chapter 1 Introduction

This book is for you if there is a soft penis somewhere in your life, and you want to be sexual in some way. Whatever the reason for your erectile differences, and whether you are solo or partnered, you are welcome here. While I often speak directly to people who have a soft penis between their legs, I also hope many partners will find value in this book.

Your soft penis is here for a reason, or a season. This book isn't about fixing erectile function, although relaxing into your softness can contribute to recovery. And it isn't really about researching how and why some penises do or don't get as hard as their owners or partners want.

It's about pathways to sexual pleasure that bring joy into your life. I'm inviting you to explore better ways of being sexual, beyond erections. Living well with that limp penis, whether it remains that way for only a short time, or for years, or perhaps for the rest of your life.

If you are reading this book then it is likely that either you or your partner, or both of you, have deep experience of the wasteland of loss when that soft, vulnerable penis is unable to transform into a firm magic wand. Yet you are here. It takes courage to experience loss and find the will to adapt.

Nothing that follows is intended to take away from the joy of erections for their owners and sex partners. Adventuring into the playground of soft penis sex need not stop you exploring pathways to erectile recovery.

But there is a lot to be gained from recasting sex in a way that is less erection dependent, and more creative, varied, loving, and involving the entire body. This also involves helping your thinking, emotions and relationships adapt to their new reality.

1.1 Medical considerations

This book is intended to be read as a supplement but not an alternative to professional medical advice. A man's penis is an extremely sensitive indicator of many things, some of which are important medical conditions. If your penis is not getting erections, or its erectile function has changed substantially, you should consult a medical doctor. I am not qualified to diagnose medical conditions that lie behind changes in your erectile function. These can include diabetes, heart disease, the impact of medications and surgery, problems with diet and exercise, and many more.

In these pages the focus is on how to have fun and connect with loving partners with your penis just the way it is. You should seek out and take professional advice both on your overall health and on possible options for strengthening erectile function.

1.2 Relationship challenges

People often call prostate cancer *the divorce disease* because it puts so much strain on intimate relationships regardless of the genders of each person. While our focus here is on erectile differences for men, remember similar challenges emerge for woman and their intimate partners during and after treatment for breast cancer.

When a person has a core part of their sexual body identity taken away, it freaks us out and, in turn, it upsets our relationships with intimate partners. In some cases, it breaks relationships.

When sex and relationships aren't working easily, many people tend to withdraw - or to lash out at their partners. It is normal to be upset, hurt, angry, sad and more. It is not okay to take that out on your partner. And while it is also okay to step back from the world and your relationships when you are hurt, withdrawal is not a good long-term strategy.

This book invites you to take stock of your intimate relationships and provides some starting points to share the process of adapting to change. But the focus here isn't on the deep work required to heal those relationships. If you do have a partner and your relationship is suffering, I encourage you to find a relationship coach or counsellor that suits you. Also, it's important to go together to any medical or therapeutic consultations regarding one partner's sexual health. You are both affected.

The most common thing I hear from men with limp dicks is "I just wish I could satisfy my partner" but I suspect the biggest problem is with the satisfaction of the penis owner himself. The good news is that you can satisfy both partners. Particularly in Chapter 3 Pleasure, you will find lots of ways to have fun with a soft penis, and even experience new forms of penetrative sex. More importantly, let your partner know that you still want them.

1.3 Recalibrating sexual signals

Once my girlfriend realised that my ED was about me and not about her, she relaxed and we were fine.
Wesley, 48, UK. Has experienced ED throughout his adult life.

If you used to get hard and now your penis remains soft in a sexual situation with your partner, they might take that as a signal that you are no longer aroused by or sexually interested in them. If you do still desire your partner sexually, then you can reduce misunderstanding by telling them out loud when you are aroused, specially when your penis is not able to show it in the old erect way.

In this sense, it is up to the owner of a soft penis to get used to his new body, and then to be mindful of how partners and potential partners might misinterpret that softness as lack of sexual interest in them.

1.4 Getting practical

While I don't shy away from the mental, emotional and energetic struggles involved, at the heart of this book is a series of practical activities and suggestions for you to explore and discover sexual pleasure in your new body, with or without a partner. Because the subject of sex including penises without erections has been so taboo for so long, there is a huge gap in literature, erotica, and both public and private conversation.

This book is here to help you and any partner(s) in your life get going – not to follow any strict recipes, but to try a few new possibilities and create your own delicious menus from there.

It's an invitation to re-imagine the possibilities of pleasure and sexual connection beyond the need for erections.

1.5 Language and sources

My reason for using some colloquial terms is simply to indicate that the intention of this book is to be down to earth. It is not academic, and the topic is an earthy one. Birth, sex and death are about as primal as one can get.

In this book I often speak directly to the person with the soft penis. We have first-line responsibility for understanding and adapting to the changes in our own bodies. And I believe there is a dearth of male voices on this subject. Everybody is equally welcome to take this book and use it, including partners and people with penises who don't identify as men.

My lived experience is as a white, cisgendered and primarily heterosexual male. The people whose voices contributed to the making of this book include all races, gender identities and sexual orientations, aged from 20s to 90s and across five continents. The book is intended to be relevant to people of any gender and sexual orientation, and whether you are in one or more intimate relationships, or dating, or single.

Every personal quotation in the text is from a real person, and used with their explicit permission. In the text, only their first name, age and country are provided as situational markers. Where further information has been published about their stories, the links are provided in the Resources section and the Readers Portal online, along with a select bibliography of books and articles.

I have tried to keep my language simple and direct. One consequence is that I'm often going to talk about the soft penis in your life as "your" penis, even though I really mean "your or your partner's penis." It can get cumbersome to repeat the words "you and your partner" throughout. Please understand that my intention is to include partners and not to confuse whose penis it is. I recognise that this stuff matters both to the person whose body the penis is attached to, and any partner or partners who might be sexually active or interested.

1.6 Accepting changes in shape

Every soft penis is okay and deserves to be loved. Each one is different. Maybe you can find one a bit like yours in this gallery:

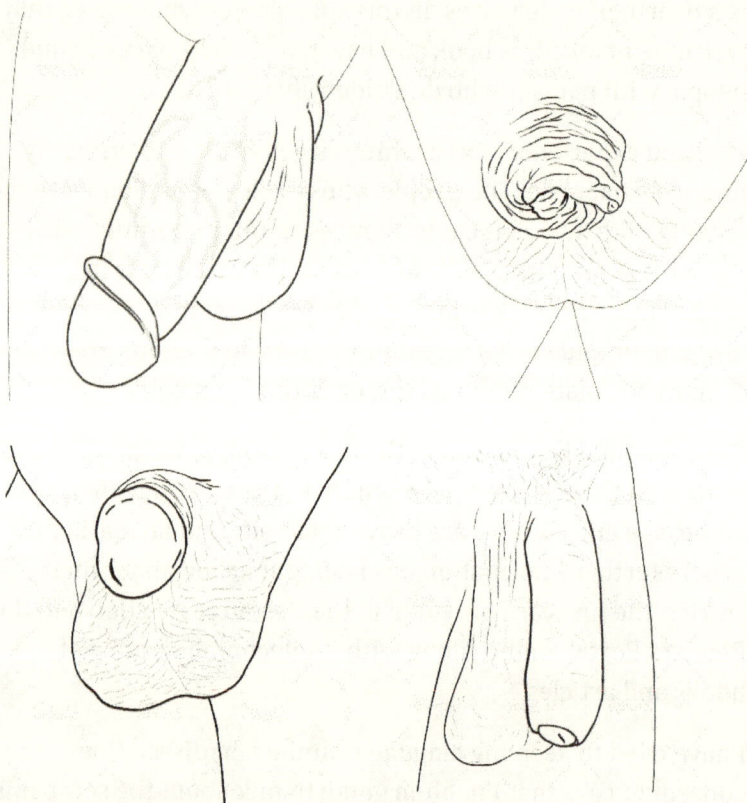

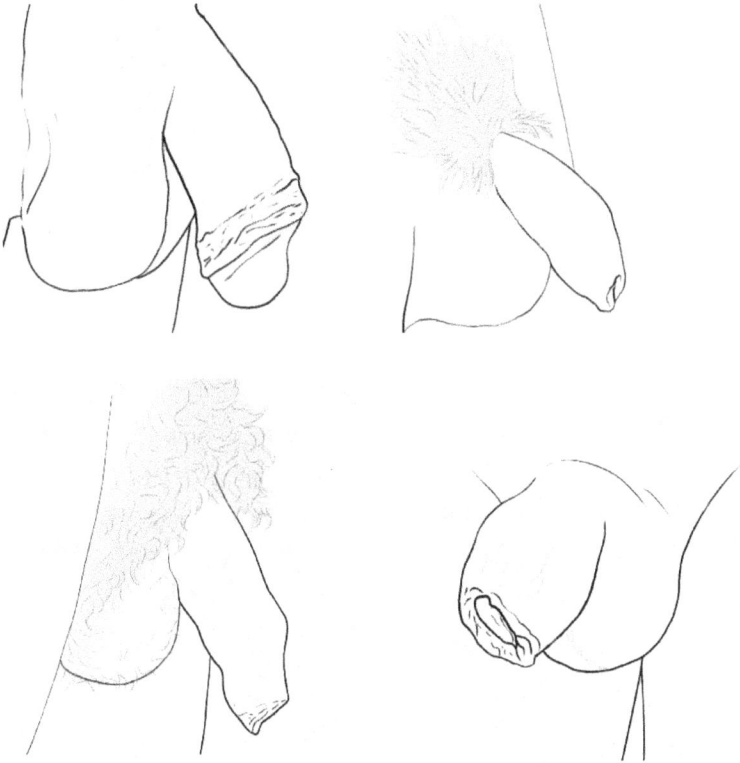

Let yourself look. It is okay. Each one of these penises has a story to tell. Each one has a way to be pleasured, and a way to be shamed. Which will you choose, shame or pleasure?

1.7 Personal stories that connect us

Each one of us is less alone than we think. The best way I know to remind us that we are not alone is to tell our own stories and listen to other people's stories.

There are lots of stories in this book and more in its companion websites, BeyondErections.com and Recoveringman.net. I have quoted contributors verbatim, in their own words. Here are milestone excerpts from the yearlong story of a US couple in their 70s slowly adapting to sex beyond erections after his prostate cancer treatment, written by the husband.

November 2023: *Getting hard, getting aroused, feeling my dick pulsate, are three things I miss incredibly. I was telling someone recently that I knew what the words, ED, meant but I really didn't understand the emotions connected to it.*

Playing with your wife and having her play with you, enjoying passionate foreplay – and having your dick lay there sound asleep is devastating. I want to pound so badly and I have nothing to pound with. My wife has even said, I need to feel you inside me and ride me real hard.

Having said all of that, I know I can be greatly relieved if I could just mentally and emotionally separate hard-ons from orgasms and sex. At this time I just don't know how to get there.

July 2024: *I lived in the 'hard or nothing' realm all my sex life and now am having to come to terms with softness. With intercourse being so much work these days we find ourselves focused on planning sex rather than having sex. And she wants to feel the fullness of my hardness inside her.*

November 2024: *My wife and I had a really nice love making time this morning! I super enjoyed having my hand on her genitals and my finger stroking her clitoris. It was fun bringing her to orgasm and I was able to roll on top of her and hump her with my soft penis. It was truly sublime humping even with a soft dick. Pressing my pelvis into hers was heavenly.*

I then did a [quadmix injection] shot and was able to give her a hard-on penetration she especially enjoyed. A good time was had by all. Hoping to meet at the

same place soon. I was only able to have one orgasm but oh what an O!"
Tom, 77, USA. No natural erections since prostate surgery.

Notice the elapsed time. This couple spent a year of trial and error between the utter despair of the opening paragraphs, and the tentative discovery of some "truly sublime" sexual pleasure with a soft penis.

1.8 Men are opening up

Being labelled with "erectile dysfunction" is terribly isolating. Once that label applied to me, I was painfully reminded how many colloquial sayings and jokes centre around men "not being able to get it up." And it's not like a broken leg which everybody can see and sympathise with you about. A broken erection is invisible except in intimate sexual situations.

Yet you are not alone if you or your partner has a soft penis. While it's difficult to get accurate global data, JB McKinlay's 2000 analysis suggests that some form of erectile dysfunction affects about half of all men over 50. This includes most of the men who are diagnosed with prostate cancer every year, estimated by the World Health Organisation at over 1.4 million per annum worldwide. Almost all of those treated will experience some form of temporary or permanent erectile dysfunction.

At first, every one of these men suffered in silence. Many relationships broke up as the man with the soft penis either withdrew or was rejected. But now there are alternatives. Every day I meet more men who are opening up about their experiences and sharing stories, like Tom in the quote above. Every time we hear about another man's struggles and explorations – including how they manage to have enjoyable sex without a firm erection – we are less alone, and we get new ideas that might help us adapt and thrive in our new bodies.

I have been lucky enough to sit in the global *Recovering Men* circle for more than four years. I am inspired by the myriad ways these men cope, support each other, and share personal experiences that in turn unlock new explorations. We meet live and on video. What they say is not included here because the conversations are confidential, but their experiences inspire this book.

Each person's journey to intimate connections with themselves, and any partner if present, is unique. Every chapter ends with some suggested activities to help you make sense of your world mentally, physical and emotionally. There are no right or wrong answers.

You have been landed in an unfamiliar place, without your usual gear. This book aims to guide, encourage and accompany you as you hunt for hidden pleasure. Beyond the wasteland of loss lies a treasure trove of joyful, playful pleasure that makes the old pump-pump-pump genital-focused sex seem one dimensional and over-simplified.

1.9 Further exploration

The path is made by walking. I invite you to try one or more of these activities, or make up another action step that suits you:

- Make a list of *hard penis* myths and sex expectations that impact you.
- Debunk some of those myths and challenge some of those expectations. You might do this in conversation with a trusted friend, or in private writing.

- Ask a close friend or partner about ways they have enjoyed sexual pleasure without an erection being required.

Chapter 2 Mindset

To enjoy sex beyond erections, the people involved often need to rewrite negative scripts about erectile differences. These might include beliefs that sex requires a hard penis, shaming of erectile differences, narrow mainstreaming of what sexual practices are acceptable, and a kind of fossilisation of ideas of what it means to be a man.

Images of erections have been linked to masculinity throughout human history. Directors of contemporary porn videos require their male stars to be hard from the moment their trousers come down till the moment the camera stops rolling.

Real life is different.

2.1 Good sex doesn't require a hard penis

According to the Oxford English Dictionary online, sex is defined as: "physical activity between two people in which they touch each other's sexual organs, and which may include sexual intercourse." There's nothing in that definition that requires a hard penis or penetrative intercourse.

But here are some of the conventional beliefs about sex that are locked into just about every movie, TV show, commercial advertisement, novel, and marital expectation on this planet. Do you recognise them?

- Sex is all about penetration. Anything else is "just foreplay."
- Men must be hard to have sex.
- Sex is the only way to intimacy.
- Sex isn't satisfying if it doesn't "finish" in orgasm.

If there is a soft penis in your life, these beliefs can be barriers to your sexual satisfaction as well as your intimate relationships.

Sex that is only about fucking is so limiting - but so easily holds the actor captive, and thereby keeps the world of sensuality far away.
Michael, 66, South Africa. Erections limited due to antidepressant medication.

In real life, sexual pleasure can be experienced and shared regardless of gender and body shape. To address those four limiting conventional beliefs in turn:

- Penetration is not a universal requirement for all good sex. There are penetration options even with a soft penis included in Chapter 3.
- Men and their partners can have mind-blowing sex without erections and the next chapter suggest some ways of getting there.
- In this book the term *intimacy* is not used as a polite name for sexual intercourse. Rather, I use the word *intimacy* to describe private physical and emotional closeness between two or more people. We can be intimate with our partners without necessarily being sexual. For some, including many on hormone-blocking androgen deprivation treatment (ADT), the best intimacy is built primarily on sensuality.

- Orgasms come in many forms, and soft penis sex often requires some adjustment which is addressed in Chapter 4. Orgasms are not necessarily the "finish" of a sexual engagement – various climaxes may occur all along the way, and also some satisfying sex might not include any conventional orgasm.

Orgasm is sometimes termed "finishing" as the expected and desired end point of a sexual encounter. I think this creates such unrealistic expectations – and not just for seniors and people who've had prostate problems. We are getting better and better at focusing on connections at all levels and of all sorts between us post-surgery, when we can't rely on a persistent erection during sex. We are finding our way to being sexual without anticipation of what may or may not happen.
Colleen, 72, Canada. Partner of author.

2.2 Unshaming erectile difference

When a penis remains soft even in sexual situations, this can attract a lot of unwelcome attention that compounds the problem. Often, either the penis owner or their partner simply withdraws. There may be shame involved. However, penises are extraordinary organs in all the shapes and forms they occur and can be a source of delight to their owners and partners regardless of shape and firmness. It just takes a while to get over the messages of sexual shame that echo around every flaccid penis.

It is time to take away the shame of erectile difference and replace it with curiosity - the curiosity of an explorer discovering how to give and receive pleasure to this astonishing bundle of tissue and nerves.

What we are doing, in unshaming and enjoying soft penises, is huge. The world is convinced that the only ways to do sex with men all involve and require hard penises. As a wise sex educator said to me,

---

Everyone sees the world through the eye of the penis, until we learn better.
Delene van Dyk, South Africa. Sex educator.

As you begin to make the shift towards a less penis-centred world, be aware that this is not just a wrench for you personally. You are affected by the social and cultural system around you that tends to disapprove of soft penises in sexual situations. You can be part of a change that is needing to happen in the wider society around you.

2.3 Different strokes for different folks

Because of the monotonous narrative about genital penetrative sex that surrounds us, it can be difficult to recognise opportunities for sensual and sexual pleasure. Sexual pleasure involving non-erect penises is rarely depicted or discussed in movies and on social media as well as in social conversation.

To widen your options, I will suggest a lot of different activities. You might consider some of them taboo, or too kinky - or not kinky enough. Like at a buffet, you can simply leave things you don't like on the table.

Many innocent and juicy pleasures lie beyond one or other boundary set up consciously or unconsciously by stories, beliefs and conventions.

Pushing back the mountains of expectation, convention and quite possibly shame is a huge and heroic task. I'm here to engage low gear with you, to find that inner earthmoving equipment we all have, to move those mountains. To illustrate the challenges, here is a personal story from my first, temporary, experience of erectile difference when I was about 50.

The first time my erections disappeared during sex it was devastating. There was a big drama going on at that time in my life about the end of a business partnership. One morning, in the middle of penetrative sex with my wife, my erection simply faded away. At first I just tried to hump harder, thrust more, in ways that had previously brought me back to full hardness. But this time it didn't help. I soon slipped out and couldn't really "point" to get back in. I felt desperate and ashamed, like millions of other men before and since then.

What was different was that my wife reached down, felt my flaccid penis, realised we couldn't continue with intercourse, and said "never mind, we can still make love."

I cried! I cried for my loss. I cried for her tenderness and understanding. Most of all I cried for the shame she released. And my heart opened up to our ongoing loving. We let my little soft sausage slide up and down the wet smooth groove of her vulva. Indeed we continued to make love.

Looking back on that period, which only lasted a few weeks, I realise how stuck I was in shameful assumptions:

- If I can't be hard then love and sex are over.

- If I can't maintain an erection during sex, I expected to be shamed by my partner.
- I was terrified the news would get out to the world that "Mish can't get it up."

I am deeply grateful for my wife's loving and wise response. So quickly and clearly, she went way beyond all of those shaming assumptions. She was truly making love in that moment, and in turn that enabled our shared lovemaking to continue. In so doing, she also helped me start building the courage which led me more than 15 years later to write this book.

Not everybody is as lucky as me.

2.4 What has been lost

Each person who once had pleasurable erections, and has now lost that capability, needs time to process their emotions about the change. Grieve your loss, mourn it. Let your emotions out! But please don't blame yourself or your partner.

This is something that has happened to you. Loss is a normal part of life. Adapting to loss is a spiritual and emotional process that takes time. Each person has their own way.

If you would like a mental framework to examine your own sense of loss the five stages of grief model might help. It was first published by psychiatrist Elisabeth Kübler-Ross in 1969, denoting the stages as denial, anger, bargaining, depression and acceptance. In practice they don't always follow in any particular order.

There is no reason that your experience needs to be shoe-horned into her framework. But it could be useful for you to ask yourself, or discuss with a trusted friend, partner, or care provider:

- What part of your experience with erectile difference are you denying, hiding or avoiding?
- What are you angry about? How can you express your anger without doing more damage to yourself and/or other people?
- Who or what might you be bargaining with, to get it all back? This could include doctors, your partner, time, physical fitness, overeating, working even harder ...
- Are you depressed? Do you possibly need professional help?
- What aspects of your current situation do you accept? What might be possible if you accepted more of what has already happened and can't unhappen?

2.5 Let go of comparison

If you compare your soft penis to your prior experience of it in full hardness, you may well be disappointed, at least at first.

Take your time. Remember how much fun you had with a hard penis. Depending on your situation, you may also want to imagine or envision how much fun you might have if and when it gets hard again.

Then let it go. Comparing with history too much can hold you back. For now at least, you have a new and different body. Your job is to turn the page, make a new plan, create a new chapter in the book of your sex life.

You sometimes get full erections, and other times stay soft in sexual situations. Comparison between those two current realities may be just as much of a distraction for you. I found that when erections first started to come back, they tended to push all other forms of sexual pleasure and interaction into the background. The thing to remind yourself is that pleasure is possible whether soft or hard. It's just different when you are soft.

2.6 Compassionate invitation

Approach everything with compassion – for this soft penis, for the body and mind it belongs to, and for any partner or partners involved. You will be sucked back into comparison from time to time. Forgive yourselves - it is both personal and systemic.

Keep the invitation open. Invite this soft penis to show itself. Invite it to feel your love. Invite it to notice what feels good to it now, in its soft state. If partners are involved, invite their compassionate loving care. Remind yourself to keep loving yourself and any partners who may be involved, and let them love you.

2.7 Sex dates

You schedule just about everything that is important to you, from a dinner date to a hike in nature, and from taking your kids to school to attending their graduation.

Now, if you weren't doing so already, it is time to consciously carve out time for sex dates. These may be with your partner or with yourself. The point is to make time where you won't be disturbed, where you can set aside distractions, and focus on sexual pleasure and intimacy.

Making dates for sex play was really helpful for us after my husband had prostate surgery and mostly had a soft penis. As we learned about his new body, the hard cock urge for lustful sex wasn't there. Having a date meant I had time, as did he, to prepare myself with ideas.

We agreed in advance that the intention was exploration, not penetration or orgasm. This gave us

permission to experiment without the previous
expectations of beginning, middle, and end. We make
a date once a week, and also play at other times as we
feel. Without the dates, I think sex play could get lost
amongst other activities and fade away.
   This is something neither of us wants to happen.
Colleen, then 69, South Africa. Partner of author.

Creating sex dates is not the end of spontaneous sex. But scheduled time is likely needed to help create the route to satisfaction for you and your partner, given the reality of your new and different body. You need time to get to know how your own body works. Your partner needs time to relearn your pleasure pathways. Your relationships need time to adapt.

A sex date might be as simple as saying "we will lay in bed a bit longer on Sunday mornings and make time for some sex play." Or it might be a special event that you prepare for well in advance. Create the right atmosphere in the location you choose for your date. You might consider appropriate music, lighting, perhaps a fire, incense, or candles, suitable cushions. Make a plan to minimise the chance of an emergency call from children or parents or other people you care for. Each prepare your own body to be delectable – wash with extra care, think about perfume, adornments, and sexy clothes or accoutrements. Or take a shower or bath together.

There are no limits – use your imagination. Design the date together, or take turns at surprising each other.

2.8 Shifting energies and eagerness

Many people find themselves almost constantly in a state of erotic arousal. The nature of male bodies and hormones makes this particularly common amongst young men. Many women are more aware of highs and lows of their sexual energies, often linked to their menstrual cycles.

If you now have a soft penis, you might look out for the way your sexual energies undulate over periods of days, weeks or even months. Getting used to these cycles can reduce the sense of abandonment that comes with the low parts of your sexual energy cycle.

After I lost my erections, I realised how, throughout my life, my erect penis was an enthusiasm role model for me. It carried the essence for me of "just go for it" with a grin. It reminded me to always be interested in new adventures. It modelled being able to shape-shift to suit a situation.

You might be missing the eagerness that erections brought to your life. In many ways they lead many men into life, into relationships, and into joy. This book invites you to reclaim your eagerness, and re-enter life, relationships and joy in your new body.

2.9 Further exploration

There is a lot to process in adjusting to a new body. You might try something from the following list:

- Write down in detail what you have lost. Include feeling words. Then tell it to the wind, or the sky, or your trusted friend, or your coach or therapist.
- Read a book or a blog, listen to a podcast or watch a video about grief and loss. If it doesn't resonate, try another.
- Write, record or make a selfie video telling the story of the fun you had with your erections in the past.
- Choose the way you are going to step into your life going forward. Consider options including courage, strength, connectedness, compassion, humour, candidness and many

more. Pick one or two that resonate for you and remind yourself of your commitment every day.

- Make a list of the things you like about your body now.

Chapter 3 Pleasure

Living in a new body, or with a partner whose body has changed in a significant way, is a big and primal change. It takes time. And sex is by nature a bit chaotic, unpredictable and experimental.

You're invited to take the following section on techniques lightly, like a menu in a new restaurant that you are visiting for the first time. Sample a few items, note the ones you do and don't like, and next time try a mix of new adventures and now-familiar delights.

You can try things out in any order, solo and/or partnered. Even if you prefer partnered sex play, I encourage you to take some private time alone learning and relearning how your new sexual body works.

This section focuses on receiving pleasure as a soft penis owner, and for many this is a big role change that takes time. But it does not mean I am advocating that you ignore your partner's body and pleasure! Remember, we are simply adding activities to your sexual pleasure menu, not subtracting anything. There is nothing to stop you continuing to please, surprise and delight your partner sexually.

3.1 Preparing to enjoy a soft penis

The part of your body that brought so much joy in its hard, erect, thrusting form has gone soft. Given how much fun it generated in the past, you and your partner might ask what to do with it now.

Once I felt I was capable of overcoming my fear of flying with a flaccid penis, I didn't want to give the ED oxygen and power any longer. My wife and I are joyfully sexual with my soft penis as it is.
Gavin, 67, South Africa. Limited erections after prostate cancer treatment.

The first thing is to make friends with this soft, sensitive, extraordinarily versatile body part. Remind yourself not to compare your soft penis with a hard erection. Be prepared to have fun without necessarily experiencing orgasm or ejaculation the way you did before.

Take a leisurely shower or bath before you start and take special care to wash everywhere including all around your genitals and ass and under your foreskin if you have one.

Just look

Treat your soft penis like something new in your life. Feel it. Notice the way it curves and wrinkles. How does it nestle against your body? Perhaps surrounded by a natural hairy bush. Perhaps, reaching out from your smooth-shaven pubic mound or huddled in a wrinkled cone close to your body. A smooth helmet over a short stem. Or turtling inside the surrounding flesh. If you can't see it, use a mirror or your camera in selfie mode to examine it from all sides.

Take some deep, slow breaths. Clear your mind of comparison. Just notice your soft penis and allow it to be itself. You might want to say some words of thanks for all the joy it has given you. You might want to commiserate for what it has lost. But always end with appreciation of what it is now. Let your brain and your eyes begin adjusting. Recognise the beauty and the possibility that lies in this softer, gentler, perhaps more hidden and still crucial part of your body.

If you found that difficult, forgive yourself. There is huge pressure on you to compare, to yearn for hardness. Not just from your own hard penis memories, but from the whole world's expectations and preconceptions about men. When you are ready to try again, let the comparisons go.

Allow yourself to see your soft penis for what it is. Notice the package that comes with it. Start recognising how your genitals nestle at the middle of your body, and let your appreciation go up, down, and around beyond just the pelvic area.

Loving touch

I encourage you to touch yourself. You might prefer your partner's touch. Everything that follows can be done by you, or your partner(s), in any combination. What matters is that whoever is touching is compassionate and open, and that you focus on loving and appreciating your own soft penis.

All I can say is that even when I don't get rock hard (which is all the time now), I still orgasm and my best orgasms are still from masturbating.
"Princess," 63, USA. Erections limited after prostate cancer.

Start with cupping this soft penis in the palm of your hand. Depending on size, you might include both penis and balls in this cupping. Don't move, don't expect anything outward to happen. Focus on the inner sensations for both soft penis or whole package and hand. Let that penis feel the warm love and support from the hand. Let the hand feel the soft power of that penis.

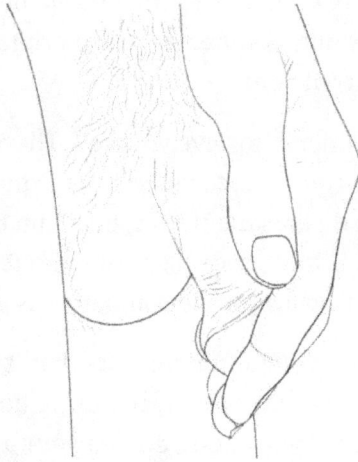

Remember – no matter how this soft penis manifests, it remains fundamentally connected to its owner's body, heart and sexual energy. It also needs the care and support of that hand. Let it feel the acceptance. Begin to feel the power oozing from this soft penis.

3.2 Taking touch further

There are so many places to go, once you have accepted this soft penis. Try to feel your own pleasure and let pleasure be your guide, going beyond erections. This applies whether you are touching yourself or you are a partner touching your loved one's penis.

Expect initial pleasure sensations to be less intense than with an erect penis. Allow yourself to sink into the sensations, whether giving or receiving or both.

Be patient. Be kind. Notice the slightest tendrils of pleasure creeping into your awareness.

Hands and fingers

Try any or all of these. As you explore, pay attention to rhythm and pace. Some parts like fast movement, others slow. Vary both pressure pulses and stroking speed and rhythm.

There is an option to try touching and stroking with and without massage oil or other forms of lubrication, provided that unlubricated touch doesn't hurt or irritate your skin. See what your new body likes now: it might have different preferences to its previous harder form.

Take your time. This is not a race. Don't expect everything to feel great. If it doesn't feel good, try it another way or simply move on to try something else. Keep your air of experimentation.

The sweetest spot just under the tip

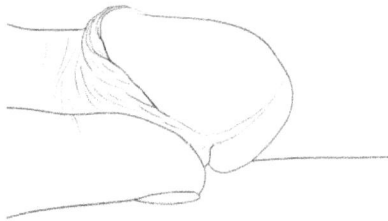

Find the sensitive frenulum on the underside of the tip, and experiment with a fingertip: how firmly does it like to be rubbed or stroked?

Where is the sweetest spot? Does it move around or remain in the same place? How fast should that finger move?

Perhaps varying pressure and pace feels good.

> *When I am very soft, I part two fingers and lay them like tramlines against my belly, with my flaccid penis flipped upwards and lying on my belly between my fingers. Then another hand or tongue can pleasure the sensitive spots without my soft cock slipping away.*
> Pedro, 64, Australia. Limited erections after prostate cancer treatment.

Exploring foreskin, if you have one

If your soft penis has a foreskin, explore the soft turtleneck tip of foreskin that protrudes beyond the head of the penis, if the skin does protrude. You might try gently rubbing it back and forth between finger and thumb.

Most foreskins really like being slowly retracted over the glans, and then back again, usually with some natural or added lubrication. Find out what makes this fun while soft.

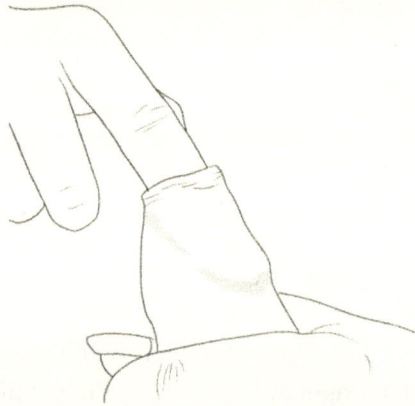

Sliding a fingertip under the foreskin may be new for you, and it's easier to do when the penis is not completely hard. You might like to experiment with this. You will need lube, whether natural or added. Fingers under foreskin can be playful and exploratory and might deliver exquisite pleasure.

Partners used to circumcised penises should be warned that an uncircumcised glans, after a lifetime of being covered by protective foreskin, is particularly sensitive.

Supportive stroking

If your soft penis is long enough to expose its own shaft, try stroking the shaft. You will likely need to support it. If your partner was used to you getting hard quickly, teach them how to hold you and stimulate you without have a hard stalk to "jack." The movement is very different. Be careful about squeezing the shaft the way you likely you used to: a firm grip with fist or tight fingers can cause a weak erection to fade.

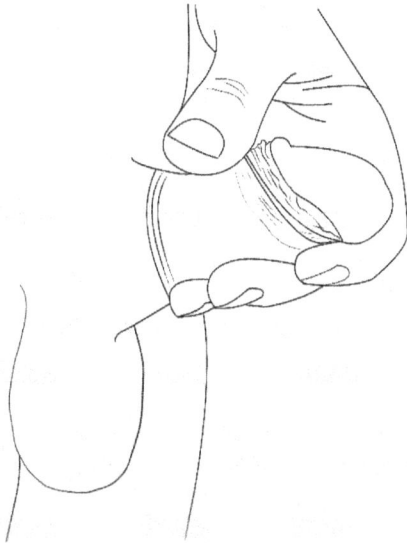

The diagram shows fingers in support rather than squeezing tightly on the shaft. At least one fingertip traverses the sensitive spots of the frenulum just under the tip.

Loving the curve

With a soft penis, it's important not to see swelling as the prelude to a hard main event but rather to enjoy and celebrate what's there.

Pay attention to the curve of the shaft. Try stroking down over the swell of the shaft, a bit like stroking down over the swell of a breast.

A new kind of "laying pipe"

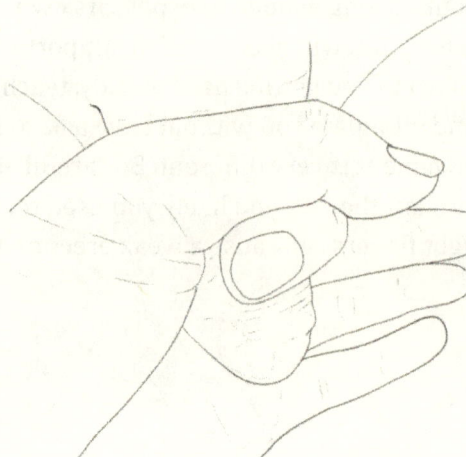

If there is any shaft exposed between base and penis head, this pipe can be loved and explored. Make a circle with thumb and forefinger and slowly slide it up and down. If the shaft isn't firm enough to support itself, you might focus on the outward stroke from base to tip.

Having the full length of a soft penis explored and stretched out like this can be extremely pleasurable. It also sometimes pushes extra blood into the head or glans area which can be fun.

Rambling around the area

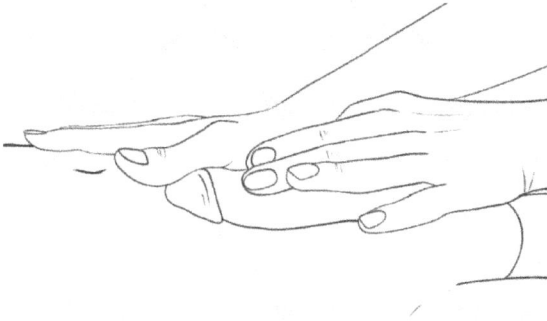

Take this soft penis on a slow and sensuous ramble around its own home ground. Roll it around. Rub it up against the belly, sideways, then down over the balls. Don't overlook this because it sounds so simple!

It is one of my absolute favourites. Seldom does a night go by without my wife cupping and fondling my soft penis and balls. We have both gotten over how soft and small it is. Instead, we pay attention to how nice it feels for both of us. We have been able to add it to the more familiar pleasure of vulva massage. It opens the loving connection between us into a torrent of energy and appreciation.

Walking naked

A very important part of your rehabilitation as a person with a soft penis is to walk naked with it. Remind yourself that your body is still a wonder of creation, even if it has other aches and pains and losses. If possible, feel the slap of your thick, soft penis against your thigh – one of the most joyful feelings for a man. Even if you think it is small and thin, feel its energetic heft.

I love to notice this in the morning, when I first get up. My "morning wood" is less like wood than rubber, but that rubbery sausage still feels glorious as it dangles and swings with intent as I get out of bed and walk naked to the bathroom.

You might like to try walking naked, side by side with your partner, each maintaining exquisite awareness of the way your own body parts dangle, rub, jiggle or swing. Build simultaneous awareness of your partner's pleasure in their own body.

Mouth, nose, cheek

Here are some options for touch that aren't just with hands.

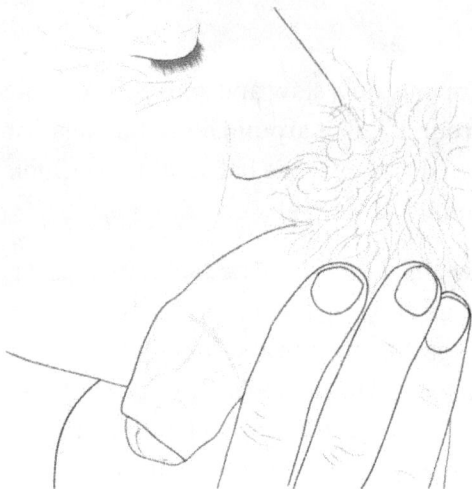

Partners, you might like to start with a nuzzle. Nosing around a soft penis can be amazing! Make sure it is as clean or musky as you like it to be before you start. Delight in the aromas and textures. Get playful as that soft penis kisses and is loved by your nose, cheeks, even ears.

I don't need to tell you to try playing with your mouth. Oral sex has been around forever and there are infinite possibilities with soft penises. What many partners like about taking a soft penis in their mouths is there is no gagging, as they can take all of it easily.

As the penis owner, you might need to get over being more passive than before. Your job in this moment is to lay back and enjoy your partner's exquisite, warm, wet and loving tongue, lips and mouth.

Remember that your own mouth can work magic all over your partner's body, whatever the state of your penis! Nothing in this section is intended to take away from the pleasure a soft penis owner can give and receive by pleasuring his partner's body.

If you are alone, explore and find out what new parts of your body are within reach of your mouth and cheeks and try some loving self-nuzzling. It can be remarkably soothing and it can be wildly erotic.

Taste, breath and nature's vibrators

Remember to pay attention to the tastes that you discover while pleasuring your partner's body with your lips, mouth and tongue. What has changed, and what has remained the same?

There are several medical conditions and treatments, including prostate cancer treatment, which drastically reduce or completely end a man's ability to ejaculate semen. That doesn't mean there's no longer anything to taste down there. While prostatectomy surgery takes away semen ejaculation, it usually leaves intact the Cowper's glands, which produce what is commonly known as pre-cum. Look out for pearly shiny clear droplets of extraordinary natural lubricant emerging from your soft, yet aroused penis. It tastes quite different to semen and is usually sweet!

Experiment with breath – where does it feel good to literally blow warm or cool streams of breath on your own or your partner's genitals? Where else does breath bring joy to your own and your partner's bodies?

Before anybody invented electric vibrators, human beings were given the ability to be a natural vibrator – in a warmer and more personal way than a sex toy can ever be. Try humming during oral sex. It's nature's first vibrator and doesn't need batteries.

Rubbing and grinding

Take time to rub your bodies against each other. Here are a few suggestions.

Thigh humping

Try rubbing your soft penis against your partner's thigh. With a bit of lube involved, you can get into some hot humping! Remember to reverse roles and have your partner rub their genitals against your thighs.

We were making dinner when my husband gave me a hug from behind, and rubbed his soft cock against me, as he passed me chopping veggies. He rubbed himself against me. It was enough for me to have a sudden lustful urge, and I asked him to stay there, and reach around into my pants. He rubbed my clit as he continued to rub himself against me for the very short time it took me to come – a welcome surprise for us both as his penis hardened as well! I'm grateful that he is happy to pleasure me without being in a specifically sexual situation, and without expecting anything in return.
Colleen, 72, Canada. Partner of author.

Full body treasure troves

Take your time to explore what other body parts feel good to rub against each other. Each human body is a treasure trove of different textures, sensations, movements and pleasures. Each idea below could be a jumping-off point to discover your own new treasures.

Tip to nip

Hold your penis against your partner's nipple and start playing. Experiment with different ways of positioning your bodies – one of you might need to kneel to get these body parts together in a comfortable way. With a soft penis, you need to have hands free, so you can both hold the penis in place and also tease and stimulate the sensitive nips and tips.

It can be extremely sexy for one partner to rub both their own and their partner's sensitive parts at the same time in this way. One or two fingertips can caress and stimulate both penis tip and nipple together. This dual stimulation can be quite sensually confusing and exciting with the different sensations and textures of your own and your partner's skin.

Crack slide

To give the penis owner more agency, try loving your partner from behind by nestling that soft penis between your partner's ass cheeks, with some lube. Slide or grind the penis back and forth in the lovely groove.

This is one form of what is sometimes called "outercourse:" both partners can thrust against each other rhythmically in a way similar to intercourse, but nobody is worrying about getting that soft penis inside the partner. The penis owner's belly and the partner's ass cheeks tend to keep the soft sausage from straying too far.

Riding without penetration

Here's a way for your partner to take charge.

Lie on your back with your softie pointing up towards your belly button. Your partner then straddles your soft penis and slides back and forth over it to delight both of you. If the top partner has a vulva, use the groove of their vulva to keep the soft penis on track and stimulate their clitoris. A couple of fingers down there can add extra stimulation to both parties as well as keeping the soft penis in position – essential if the partner on top is a man.

My wife will have me laying down on my front and slide on my ass. Then she turns me over and comes to orgasm rubbing herself up and down across my cock. NB, 63, UK. Erectile differences due to medication for enlarged prostate.

This is another form of outercourse that works well with your partner on top, and it doesn't matter how small the soft penis is. However it takes strong thighs for the straddling partner. It can get really hot, specially as that soft penis rubs against your partner's most sensitive sexual parts.

Tip to clit: less humping, exquisite pleasure
There is a wonderland waiting for you in a form of "scissoring" together, enabling both partners to find joy in the intensely concentrated bundling of pleasure nerves in the tips of your soft penis and your partner's clitoris or penis.

It's also a side-by-side position facilitating shared leadership in the sexual play.

This method works particularly well if your soft penis is small, as it doesn't require any shaft length or firmness. It also doesn't need any of the athletic strength and takes less flexibility than the straddling position described above.

If your partner is a woman, intertwine your legs together so that your soft penis nestles against her clitoris. Get comfortable and then stimulate the two sensitive tips – penis and clitoris – with one or both partners' fingertips. Make sure there is enough lubrication, adding saliva or external lube to keep everything moist and slippery.

I don't recommend a lot of humping, or the soft penis will slip out of position. Rather use fingertips to play around the soft sausage and folds and sensitive nubs. It took me a while to get over the reduced amount of humping – it taught me how wired I was for sexual thrusting.

It can be mind-blowing to feel your own or your partner's fingers wander through the pleasure maze that is created when a soft and happy penis and an excited clitoris meet in the garden of a vulva. You never know quite who is pleasing whom, and the pleasure bounces between having your genitals touched, and touching your partner's genitals.

If your partner has a penis, then the technical term for this is "frotting" but the same considerations apply: putting those two sensitive penises together, and using hands to keep them in contact with each other. You might need to slow things down a bit in honour of the needs of the soft penis. Then you can both enjoy the exquisite pleasures of putting your and your partner's most sensitive genital spots together and loving them.

3.3 Penetrating with a soft penis

Penetration of your partner with a soft penis is possible if it has a bit of semi-erect chubbiness, sometimes called a semi. In other words, if your penis is firm enough and long enough to have a discernable shaft. You need at least two inches/five centimetres of penis protruding beyond its surrounding pubis and belly. The penis doesn't need to be anything near rock hard. Nor does it need to be upright or even point in any particular direction.

Let's start with soft penis vaginal penetration. Remember the goal is to make a special connection with your partner, not necessarily to thrust and pound like you might have done before.

Regardless of position, you need lots of lube and even more patience. Willingness to play is essential – be prepared for the soft penis to slip out not just once but many times.

Body arrangement to ease soft penetration

For partners who are not so flexible or athletic, here is a position that is particularly easy and undemanding. It's a kind of scissoring. She lies on her back, legs slightly apart, near leg bent and far leg flat on the bed. He lies facing her from the side, his bottom thigh against her butt, his upper thigh under her near leg and over her far leg.

You can also try soft penis penetration in other positions of your choice including the missionary position, spooning and more.

Helping a small soft penis into a welcoming vagina

This is for a soft penis between at least two inches/five centimetres in length. Reach down, wrap part of the hand around the soft penis while pointing one finger in the direction of the welcoming vagina. Insert that finger along with the penis tip into the vagina, both making way in the entrance of the vagina and helping the soft penis along.

Don't try thrusting in such a situation. Just be glad you are connected, and let both partners savour the intimacy.

Helping a medium soft penis into a welcoming vagina

With a soft penis that is a bit longer, say four inches/ten centimetres long, either penis owner or partner can use a hand as a kind of collar around the bendy middle of the penis. Point the tip of the semi-hard penis at the well-lubricated and relaxed vagina entrance, and let the penis owner thrust gently. The hand that is collaring the body of the penis stops it from bending double.

With a push forward from the base of the penis, a collaring hand stopping it from bending too much, and a welcoming vaginal entrance in front – well, forwards and inwards is the only way to go.

Soft penetration allows us to return to our regular afternoon delights. Eight months after my husband's cystoprostatectomy, we are able to reconnect sexually without fussing too much about how hard his erections are. Our message: do not wait for correct erection to try penetration. A penis feels much better in the place where he is intended to be than anywhere else!
Catherine, 59, France. Partner lost erectile function after surgery.

For many people, the experience of re-entering their lover's vagina with their penis after a long period of ED-enforced absence is ecstatic, "almost like losing your virginity all over again" as one person described it. And this pleasure can sometimes induce a little further swelling of the penis, enough to keep the pleasure going.

Helping a soft penis into a welcoming ass

For anal penetration, it takes a very well prepared and relaxed anus and a relatively firmer soft penis, but the same methods described above can and do work. And there are other ways as outlined in the following quote.

I love to mix oral sex with rimming. I use my tongue to penetrate my boyfriend after licking all around his dick and anus and between his thighs. Even though I often can't get erections I am giving him pleasure and that is a reward in itself.
Michael, 66, South Africa. Erections limited due to antidepressant medication.

3.4 Expanding your erotic landscape

There may be erotic opportunities that either one or both of you have considered but abandoned because you are too embarrassed to ask or try, or because they just seem weird or awkward.

Now your body is demanding change. You have the opportunity to explore new or existing pathways to pleasure. Maybe you and your partner might be overlooking, or judging to be taboo, shameful or inaccessible.

I am single, age 64, I am no longer able to get natural erections but that has not stopped me from actively dating women. My partners are of a similar age to me and for some of them, due to common post menopausal reasons, penetrative sex can be uncomfortable and painful.

Faced with erectile dysfunction arising from my prostatectomy, I have had to modify my expectations of what sexual pleasure is for me and my partner. Gratification for me these days does not necessarily mean penetration and orgasm, as I can achieve great satisfaction from skin on skin, caresses, and giving pleasure through oral sex.

If you are dating without a prostate, start with a general conversation about your health issues. Remember, good relationships are not just about whether penetrative sex is possible, its about connection with and respect for each other.

Pedro, 64, Australia. Recovering from prostate cancer.

Your can find all the pleasure in both of your bodies and your relationship and bring it to the fore, without expecting or relying on your penis being a penetrator.

Oral sex

It's important not to overlook the obvious: there is nothing about your new body that precludes joyful oral sex. Consider the example of an older couple after more than ten years without natural erections. They say that his prostate cancer revitalised their sex life and his relatively soft penis makes oral sex easier for her.

Sex in our 80s keeps my wife and me young in many senses.

For oral sex we get into the 69 position so that while she gives me oral sex, I stimulate her. This is great because I tease her clitoris until she can't wait. This is new for us and it is a fantastic experience for us both.

> *I can use the [penis] pump to control the size of my erect penis to suit her, because my full erection is uncomfortable for her to accommodate.*
> Pratap, 86, UK. No natural erections since prostate cancer treatment.

You can continue to please each other with your mouths. There is no need to stop just because one of you has a soft penis. Delight in your partner's orgasms. Look for ways to enjoy the smaller size and flexibility of the soft penis. It still has the same number of nerve endings, only now concentrated into a smaller package.

Bellies

How much attention to you pay to your own and your partner's belly? Whether it is flat or curved, firm or soft, large or small it can be far more of a turn-on than many people realise.

I have discovered way more belly pleasure since my sex life expanded beyond erections. I have also realised the huge role my belly pressing against my partner's belly or ass plays in the thrills of both penetrative sex and the non-penetrative outercourse options outlined above. There is something hugely erotic for me about my core sexual energy and desire radiating out through my belly from my sex chakra buried deep inside.

Next time you press against your lover, try paying attention to the way you can penetrate them from your belly, radiating your love and lust and desire through your core and into your partner. If you or your partner's belly is large, you might need to do this lying in spooning position on your sides. If your partner is open to this, you might discover a whole lot of pleasure from fondling their belly, stroking and cupping it and feeling the power of that sexual core within.

Mutual masturbation

In addition to touching each other, there is great value in each touching yourselves while you are together. You might do this simultaneously or take turns. Self pleasuring in front of your lover is deeply revealing and empowering and may ask you to let go of shame or inhibitions you didn't even know you had. If you haven't done this for a while, it is a really important practice for both partners.

Watching your lover pleasure themself in front of you, without joining in, can bring extraordinary emotional intensity as well as being profoundly informative about what your partner really likes.

Testicles

A surprising number of men and their partners don't play much with those two lovely, delicate egg-shaped testicles that create the essence of male reproductive capacity. Playing with your balls is way underrated, particularly by straight men. Your erectile changes might be just the invitation you need to discover or rediscover a wonderful form of ballgame.

Partners may need to be reminded how sensitive testicles are to being squeezed too hard. But it is easy to start gentle and learn fast – simply have your partner gently play and let them know when it is on the edge of hurting. Keep communicating as your partner and you identify your pleasure points and possibly even a level of pain that is pleasurable for you.

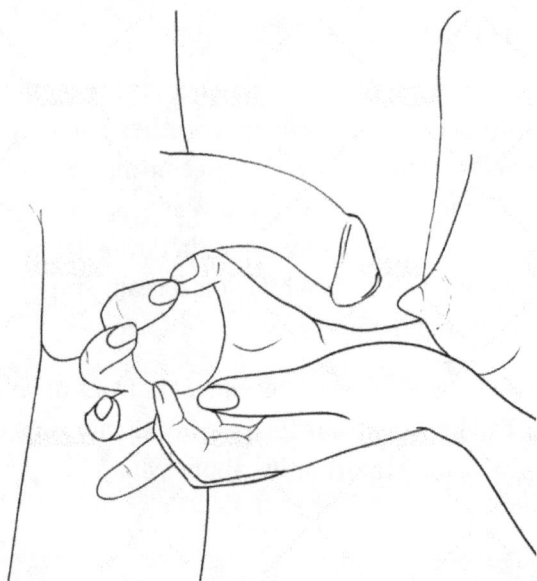

It can feel really good to use thumb and forefinger to encircle the scrotum between the body and the testicles and gently tug downwards on the whole sac. It feels different at different levels of arousal, so remember to try it both as an early part of foreplay and during maximum arousal.

It gets a bit more intimate when a partner handles individual testicles with fingers, lips and/or tongue. There are lots of personal preferences to explore here. Do each of you have preferences for natural pubic hair or shaved genitals? For many, being fresh and clean is an absolute must. For others a bit of masculine muskiness is an added turn-on that they prefer not to wash away before playing.

Having grown up a boy in a boy's school, I recognise that the whole idea of testicles being an erotic source of pleasure was completely foreign to me. The narrative amongst boys growing up in my time was all negative, including being kicked in the balls and the fear of having one's balls grabbed and squeezed or crushed. If any of this legacy has affected you or your partner, you might like to name it, shake it off, and begin all over again.

Your testicles are a gift, and their importance and pleasure can spread way beyond their role in reproduction.

Perineum (Taint)

The strip of flesh between scrotum or vulva and anus is a wonderful playground for all genders. It is technically called the perineum but some people call it the taint. I encourage you to explore all kinds of touch and play in this area, including deep massage. Depending on your kinks it can get either dangerously or enticingly close to forbidden zones but don't let that stop you exploring.

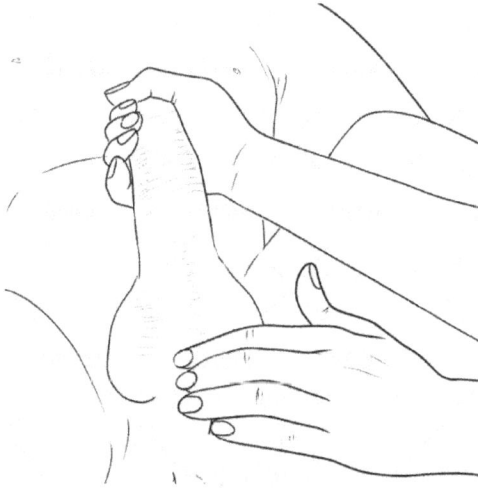

For people with prostates, pay attention to the deep reverberations as you massage over what is often called "the P spot." P is for prostate which is indeed a glorious nubbin of joy. And even after surgical removal of the prostate in cancer treatment, the same area remains delightful for many men.

Armpits

Who finds armpits sexy? I used to love rubbing my erect penis in my partner's armpits. Perhaps you can explore what erotic delights emerge from the feelings, smells and textures of armpits with or without body hair in either yourself or your partner.

Anal play (without involving a penis)

As mentioned earlier, there is a huge variety of anal play to explore if you are open to that. There are very real hygiene considerations about anal play, so you need to wash the area well before playing, and be sure that you don't use the same toy or body part to penetrate other orifices once it has been involved in anal play, without washing.

I have a vibrator I use for anal pleasure. When I feel ready to take it in, I generally lay still, almost motionless and try to relax and sense the vibrations. As my pelvis relaxes my back arches. The vibrator and the vibrations seem to expand out into the bowl of the pelvis. With slow motions and paying attention the whole area becomes more excited and I move into the dance of tension and relaxion. The vibrations seem to produce small peaks of erotic energy in my bladder, chest and nipples, my lips and hips. What had started as sensual has now become erotic and my mind and breath have become more involved. Sometimes porn that I have watched appears in my mind but I generally try to refocus on what I am experiencing in the moment. I love when my nipples become hot and sensitive and my ass arches enough to know it has been felt and filled. Sometimes my penis becomes a little firmer and I can feel sensations in my balls. I

discover what in the moment this body is willing to allow and how to support that naturally and lovingly and joyfully.
Adrian, 69, USA. Unable to get full erections.

Here are some exciting anal possibilities that don't require you to have an erection:

- Going from palming your partner's ass cheeks to fingering closer and closer to their anus can be super exciting particularly if you take your time, edging closer and closer and feeling into both partners' comfort and pleasure.
- Set a hygiene standard that both partners are comfortable with and keep to it.
- Just a fingertip with some lube playing around the anal ring and carefully, gently penetrating as far as the first knuckle is a great way to take anal play internal without any pain. It's also easy to quickly and easily back off if either partner is uncomfortable. And it is a great way of enjoying solo play. It's convenient to explore in the shower where hygiene is easy.
- Don't rush yourself or your partner. If and when you are ready, you might like to try pushing that finger further in, adding a second finger, or introducing a toy.

I find receiving any kind of loving anal penetration simply delightful. Just being touched around the outside is almost as richly erotic as the most sensitive parts of my penis – and there is the thrill of something a bit taboo beginning to happen. Then the sensation of actually being entered – whether with a toy or a fingertip or anything else – is sensual, fulfilling and explosively exciting.

Men receiving penetration

There is something primal and deeply satisfying about both fucking and being fucked.

It's that simple, and that's why I also used the crude term *fuck*. It carries the ancient resonance of urgency, lust, abandon, desire, messiness, sweat and passion. And if your previous sexual go-to was pushing your hard penis into somebody else's orifice(s) then I don't need to tell you that your soft penis has cut you off from something wonderful.

What might be worth waking up to, though, is the possibility of the penetration going the other way. There is no questioning the fact that your mouth and your anus are orifices with gazillions of pleasurable nerve endings, that can be penetrated in a variety of ways. What is in question is whether you and your partner would like to explore these options. I encourage you to at least talk about it. Maybe you will decide to try some additional steps beyond the previous section.

Being penetrated anally requires some preparation, particularly when this is a new experience for the receiver. You might benefit from consulting a detailed guide. There are examples in the resources section of this book. For now, here are some tips:

- Go very slowly, especially for the first few times you try.
- Be open to find pleasure wherever it comes, including the outer skin surrounding your anus, the anal ring itself (first knuckle of finger penetration), and the possibility of deeper penetration. There is a whole second level of penetration beyond about five inches/13 centimetres inside your rectum which only a portion of anal players enjoy.
- Once you have found your comfort level in terms of girth and depth of penetration, you might like to explore varying pace and vigour of movement.

- Men with prostates can get extra pleasure from anal stimulation, but people without prostates including men after prostate surgery can still get orgasmic levels of anal sexual pleasure.
- Most people carry a lot of emotional energy stored up in every intimate orifice. If this is the first time anybody penetrates your anus in a loving way, expect strong emotions. Welcome them and give yourselves time and space to let those emotions flow before you try to get too sexually active.

For some, being penetrated anally can bring back the same or even higher levels of passionate fucking pleasure as they had when their own penises were hard enough to do the deed. It doesn't matter what gender your partner is – partners without penises can wear a harness with a strap-on dildo as detailed below. You can also penetrate yourself solo with finger(s) or a dildo. If you find you like anal play, a world of pleasure awaits you.

Who's active and who is more passive?

Men often play the role of initiator in sexual situations. There is something about erections that seems to encourage men to be active, driving, thrusting. A soft penis invites its owner and partner(s) to explore role changes. We have already talked about owners of soft penises learning to lay back and enjoy being pleasured. Don't forget these alternatives as well:

- You might make the pleasuring completely one-way just for a while. By agreement between partners, you can set aside time where one person is solely responsible for pleasuring the other. Later you can switch roles and repeat. This can be liberating, sexy, and uncover new erotic potential in both partners. It might include having the one who is giving pleasure keep their clothes on, just for a change.

- You can try exaggerating the role reversal. This might include one or both partners cross-dressing.

3.5 Toys, medicines and other non-human helpers

This book focuses on natural sexual pleasure with erectile differences, without requiring medication or mechanical help. However, you might include or consider including toys or professionally advised medical interventions that suit your situation.

These are summarised here for your convenience and as a brief introduction to a vast array of options. See a doctor regarding any medical interventions. For easy access to non-medical resources including personal stories and reviews from users of a variety of sex aids, please visit the online Readers Portal for this book.

New inspiration might come from an in-person visit to a good quality sex store, with your partner if you have one. Consider whether you both prefer a place that is tasteful and well-lit, or you might be drawn to something with a touch of sleaze. It's important that it is sex positive. In most such stores, the staff are both discreet and disarmingly candid. If you choose to discuss your needs with them or ask a few questions, expect simple, non-judgemental and very practical answers, and no shaming whatever you might ask about.

Something similar applies to online stores. You might prefer to conduct online searches in what your browser calls incognito mode which keeps your sexual interests a little more private. Also, be aware that online searches for sex toys often throw up some crude and brash advertising offerings. You may choose to navigate past these to find rich and infinitely varied options that stimulate your senses and your imagination.

Vibrators

Vibrators are probably the easiest pleasure-based helpers to coax a soft penis to get a little firmer and make orgasms more likely, with the benefit that both partners can enjoy the vibrations with bodies entwined. What matters is that you experiment to find the shape, size, power and style that works for you. If you haven't tried vibrators for a while, or stuck only to the cheapest options, please be aware that there are now a vast array of vibrating toys designed for individuals and couples.

I started to like vibrators when I discovered the more powerful, rumbly type. Personally, I don't like the cheap fast buzzy bullet vibrators. But there is no right and wrong here.

Penis rings

If you are able to get partial erections, penis rings are a brilliant way to get them a little firmer and keep them lasting longer. A constriction ring around the base of the penis helps to stop blood from exiting the penis. It traps whatever blood your body manages to send into your penis and builds up a bit more pressure. You will need to experiment to find the shape and size that works for you, and honour the time limits on wearing a ring (often no more than 30 minutes for health reasons).

Penis pumps – vacuum erection devices

Vacuum erectile devices (VEDs) are amazing for penile rehabilitation after prostate surgery, and at any stage if you are not able to get erections at all or only very weak erections. Essentially, VEDs enable you to pump up an erection in almost any flaccid penis without any medication, provided you can tolerate the mechanical discomfort. The best pumps are well integrated with a constriction ring you can leave at the base of the penis to retain the blood once it is fully engorged.

These pumps don't have to be restricted to medical rehab. When I first got a VED I was stunned and overjoyed to be reunited with my old friend – the trusty erection that had been an almost constant source of joy and erotic connection for the previous 50 years of my life.

After practicing alone with a penis pump I began to wonder if it might help my wife and me return to penetrative intercourse. It took me weeks to pluck up the courage to suggest it, fearing she would find it unsexy and distracting. I was pleasantly surprised by her response.

"I'm used to awkwardness and planning for good sex," she said matter-of-factly. "Remember when we were young and I used a diaphragm for birth control? That was awkward and messy. Remember the times we were hot and impatient, and I was trying to insert the four inch/ten centimetre springy diaphragm into my vagina, lube all over the place, and it slipped out of my fingers and slingshotted across our bed like a frisbee? As a woman, I know about awkward preparation for sex and it is all OK."

With this encouragement, next time we had a sex date, I brought the pump to bed. She was quite curious about how it worked, and marvelled at the way my penis grew in front of her eyes. It took several attempts and we had to laugh a lot at the mess. But eventually we both enjoyed using the VED to bring back penetrative sex onto our sexual menu.

You might like to try using a pump and bringing it into the bedroom as part of your new and deliciously varied sex life.

Strap-ons (for him and her)

Here is one man's story of his journey to wearing a strap-on prosthetic dildo for heterosexual intercourse. At the time he was in his 50s and on long term hormone suppression treatment, known as androgen deprivation therapy (ADT). This extract is in the man's own words as recorded in a peer-reviewed academic research paper.

I imagined that sex performed with such an appliance would be wholly contrived and not a sensual act at all... I had never used sex toys. I was afraid that I would feel foolish and humiliated by using a strap-on penis.

Despite my reservations, I eventually agreed to experiment with a strap-on dildo. My expectations, though, were muted. At most, I thought I might be able to please my partner. But I honestly did not envision recreating a fully satisfying sexual experience....

Before this purchase, I discussed extensively with my partner ... She was at first hesitant but ultimately supportive of the exploration. We have now used the dildo many times. It caught me by total surprise how natural intercourse felt with this strap-on device. I discovered that my hip movements with the dildo on were the same as during normal intercourse. Our body contact and embrace was full and natural, as well.

KM Warkentin et al, Journal of Sex & Marital Therapy, 2006.

It is amazing how deeply personal, intimate, and exciting, it can be to give and receive penetrative intercourse using a strap-on dildo.

Penis owner wearing strap-on dildo

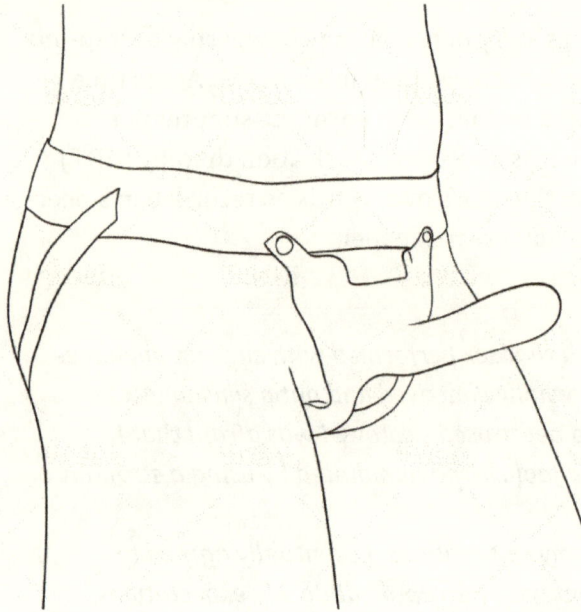

This allows you to have intercourse, penetrating your partner much the way you used to. Your bodies' basic sexual movements and rhythms can continue in the ancient way.

There are two types, the first of which is hollow, shown below. Your soft penis is encased in a firmer, larger hollow penile prosthesis. Cool designs include very stimulating silicone sleeve interiors that can be a big turn-on for the soft penis inside.

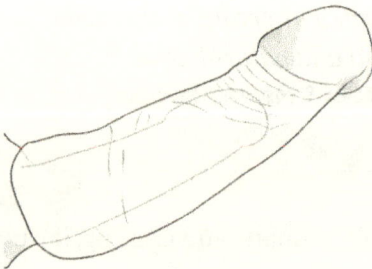

The whole contraption is held in place with a harness around your hips. Once it is comfortably fitted in place, you can penetrate your partner as if you had a hard penis, while still having your lubricated soft penis getting stimulated inside the prosthesis.

The second type of strap on dildo isn't hollow, leaving your soft penis open to manual touch as described in the story of the man on ADT which is concluded below.

The first time that [I wore the strap-on] dildo, my partner reached down and held my penis in her hand. She had coated her hand with the same lubricant used to coat the dildo and stimulated my penis in synchrony with my pelvic movements. There was little sensory difference between this act and intercourse— my penis was not in her vagina but it did not know that. It was in a wet, warm place being firmly mechanically stimulated. My hindbrain took over, and I carried the act through to orgasm, to the sexual satisfaction of both my partner and myself... If anything, sexual satisfaction has become easier, because both of us have come to accept the dildo as part of our sex play. Each time we use it, it becomes further imbued with the knowledge of the previous sexual satisfaction it has provided. It is thus now both a normal and at the same time erotic part of our lives. KM Warkentin et al, 2006.

Partner wearing a strap-on, or using double-ended dildo
The possibilities for a man opening up to receive penetration were discussed earlier. The big benefit from my perspective is that penetration still happens, there is the opportunity for

strong fucking movements, and it is a whole new experience for a man to be in a receptive role in this way.

For those who like penetration to go both ways at the same time, there is a huge variety of double-ended dildos, where each partner can insert an end in the orifice of their choice. For extra stability, most of them also work in harnesses, similar to the one above.

"Erection pills" like Viagra, Cialis and Levitra

> *"these treatment options only provide symptomatic relief in select patients."*
> Mustafa Usta et al, International Journal of Impotence Research, 2019.

Little blue pills and other generics (collectively known as PDE5i drugs) are medical magic for some people, and they simply don't work well enough for others. I'm presuming you are reading this book because the medical magic didn't completely do it for you.

If you are able to tolerate the drugs, and/or they work for you sometimes, enjoy using them to support a harder penis when you can!

> *For me, ED drugs weren't the solution, but they're very much part of the solution. Once I found the drug/dose combo that worked best, I focused on establishing "muscle-memory" of how the new erection felt. With practice, I was able to employ that memory to achieve erections without the drug.*
> Andrew, 69, Australia. 13 years since prostate cancer surgery.

Even if you find they are not working for you at present, it may be worthwhile to return to these drugs from time to time:

- Check if the effectiveness of the drugs has changed for you. As your erectile function changes, and your body changes, you might find Viagra, Cialis or Levitra or their generic alternatives working for you.
- From time to time, check if there are new formulations that work better for you. At time of writing this book some of the emergent formulations include:
  - Combining two or more of the above drugs in a single medication.
  - Faster acting formulations administered as creams, chewy gummies and more.
  - Ongoing research into drugs with less troublesome side effects.

Injections

For those willing to inject their penises just before engaging in sexual intercourse, injectable drugs often known as *Bimix*, *Trimix* and *Quadmix* can create hard erections that pop up without prior sexual arousal and last independently for several hours. I encourage you to try this without relying on it. It's just as important not to hinge your entire sex life on regaining a hard penis, as it is to grab any opportunity to have fun with an erection however you come to get it.

Implants

A long term surgical option is to have inflatable prosthetic chambers implanted in the penis, with a valve and pump for inflation positioned inside the scrotum. Many men have been deeply satisfied, and others disappointed.

I can get erections on demand. I feel no pressure during lovemaking. My erections are thicker, but my penis is the same length as before. During intercourse my penis is much more sensitive and my climaxes are much better than before.

Johann, 71, South Africa. No erections from age 57, received surgical penile prosthesis aged 68.

3.6 Further exploration

This chapter laid out a buffet of sexual options and opportunities for improvisation. It's important for you to be active in experimenting to find out what you like. Here are some suggestions to spark further exploration:

- Clear some real free time where you set aside all work completely for more than two days. Get out of doors and do whatever helps you relax. Then return to the buffet of opportunities described above. Many people find that vacations improve their sex lives.
- Repeat your favourite activity from this chapter as if it is the main event. Give up all thoughts about orgasm or hardness for yourself, and just luxuriate in the pleasure sensations. If you have a partner who orgasms treat that as a bonus but not a requirement.
- However you experienced this chapter, go back and try it another way. If you just read it, go back and try some of the activities. If you tried the activities solo, ask your partner to try some with you. If you tried the activities with your partner, make some private "me" time and try them solo.
- Explore different tactile approaches. If you tried with lots of lube, try some touch without lube or with a different type (saliva is less slippery than most modern sexual lubricants). If you normally shave body hair, try growing it out. If you

normally go natural and bushy, you might consider shaving it off.

- Download the *Exploration Possibilities List* from the **Beyond Erections** Readers Portal. It's a convenient way for you and your partner to reflect on which activities you might like to try. Each of you can go through and mark each activity with a Yes, No or Maybe according to your own preferences and curiosities. Afterwards, you can share your marked-up lists, and discuss what new things you might both be willing to try. Perhaps it will help if each of you expresses what might need to happen to make you comfortable to venture into your "maybe" zone and expand your repertoire. It's a good idea to repeat the exercise three to six months later.

- Play the two minute game, which I heard about from Tess Deveze and downloaded from Curious Creatures:

Work out who's Player One, and who's Player Two. Player Two starts a two-minute timer on their phone. Player One asks for what they want, and if need be, a quick negotiation is had, to make sure both players are happy with the request (which is how consent is built in). Once you've reached an agreement, you start [doing what they asked for], and that's what happens for the remainder of the [2 minutes]. When the buzzer goes off, you swap over, and repeat.

Roger Butler, Curious Creatures website.

- Ask what your partner finds sexy about your body, as it is now, without an erection.

Chapter 4 Satisfaction

This chapter is about how you work with your sexual energy in a new body. Men with erectile differences often find orgasms more elusive, or different.

The purpose of this chapter is to explore ways to sustain arousal and experience orgasmic climaxes throughout your whole body, without requiring erections, and to achieve full sexual satisfaction in your new body and in relationship with your intimate sexual partner.

It seems to me that sensuality and eroticism allow for much more pleasure, especially taken slowly, than lust itself. Lust is almost like a spice like chili pepper added to a meal to give it a kick, but the meal itself takes time to compose itself, cook and develop flavors before it is truly ready to eat, involving all the senses in the process of composing itself. Lust is very hard to control, in an energy sense. But even in a soft sexual encounter one can let go enough to fully experience the bliss of orgasm.
Adrian, 69, USA. Unable to get full erections.

Along the way, it's worthwhile to examine different kinds of sex, different kinds of orgasm, lust and satisfaction.

4.1 Erotic imagination

In the candid conversations I've had around the world as part of my research for this book, what I have learned about people's erotic imagination has surprised me. Far wilder sexual imagination and behaviour carries on just out of sight, or at least out of awareness of others, than you would think based on the calm exteriors most people present. Some people get off in public.

Far more people than you think are being sexual every minute of the day – in their imagination, under their clothes, just out of your line of sight. And the world is just beginning to realise how many people remain erotically active into their seventies, eighties, and even nineties.

Where does your erotic imagination go, and where might it go next, if you allow it?

Images, stories and erotic imagination

This is about going beyond porn, or behind the back of porn, or subverting porn. I think that mainstream porn is so boringly dominated by fast-and-hard sexual conventions that it does us all a disservice. It is particularly problematic for those of us with soft penises in our lives.

What is more helpful than you think (and if you are under 45 you probably already know this) is to take erotic photos and share them with just yourself and/or your partner. For many people, there is a new pathway to arousal from seeing images of your own body and your lover's and the way they entwine.

You are just as sexy as the airbrushed images online, and much more real. If this appeals, try some basic snaps. You may want to take some time to practice, get the lighting right, and move your phone around till the camera really gets a good angle. Try video and still shots.

For some people, the erotic energy is enhanced by either dressing up in new ways, or talking to each other in ways you both find sexy. Some people refer to it as talking dirty.

If you take selfie photos or videos, please take extra special care about where the images end up in world where online sharing is ubiquitous. For many people, keeping your intimate images strictly private is best and you need to be rigorous in keeping them separate from online feeds. But if everybody in the pictures fully consents, there is nothing wrong with the exhibitionism of sharing images amongst consenting adults. If you share erotic soft penis images you will be doing the world a service by shifting the dominance of the hard penis narrative. But don't even think of sharing photos or videos without your partner's full and enthusiastic consent.

I love reading erotic stories, and I particularly love them when I am struggling with my own body's limpness. My mind can go anywhere while I am reading a story.

It rots the sense in the head! It kills imagination dead!
Television, poem in **Charlie and the Chocolate Factory**
by Roald Dahl (1964)

There is something about reading that, as Roald Dahl famously said, stretches the imagination in a way that movies and photos simply can't. Images show you something, stories invite you to create something in your imagination.

This is an invitation to read erotic stories and write your own. If you have a partner, you might invite them to do it too. Share your favourite stories by reading or telling them out loud.

Finding the erotic in everyday life

Notice what is erotic for you about the world around you, particularly the natural world. Some people are turned on by being in nature. Some people are turned on by bodily functions like running, walking, exercising, or peeing. Art and architecture can both be deeply sensual. Food can be orgasmic! Social conversation can be a turn-on with or without flirtation.

For a man with a soft penis, it is a big gift to reclaim the sexiness of your own whole body. Not just your sexual parts, but the whole way you manifest in the world. Remember that different people will like different parts of you – your ass, your thighs, your shoulders, your feet, your jawline, your lips, your smile ... the list goes on and on.

4.2 Energy circuits fuel sensual lovemaking

As mentioned at the end of the last chapter, it can be enormously liberating to treat each and every form of soft penis sex not as foreplay but as the main event. Once you really give yourself and your partner permission to enjoy sex beyond erections, all kinds of joys may begin to trickle into your awareness.

Try to slow down enough to feel the subtler energies that flow when you make love in this way. The fact that "wham-bam" fast penetrative sex has been taken off your current menu might give you time to discover delightful but less obvious joys moving throughout your body throughout a variety of sexual activity.

Internal energy circuits

While pleasuring yourself, consciously follow your sensations and arousal around your whole body. There are many words that might describe what you are tracking: the zing of arousal, the pulsing of blood, the quickening of breath, prickling of skin – what are some of your signals? Include what happens below the surface, in the core of your body. For example, having your nipples stimulated might feel like there is an electric charge flowing inside your torso, down to your genitals or your belly or your toes.

Ejaculatory orgasms are very graphic in drawing attention to what spurts out of your body at climax. Ejaculating out of an erect penis can be such a powerful experience that the rest of its owner's body gets forgotten or lost. My invitation is to pay attention to the energetic fountain your penis can generate whether it is erect or orgasmic or not. This may sound a bit esoteric but it is a rewarding way to direct your attention.

Allow yourself to feel into the way sexual energy, sensation or awareness circulates around your body. Don't stress if you simply don't feel it clearly or quickly. While masturbating, some people feel an energy circuit flow from their hearts, out through their arms to their hands and fingers, into the genitals they touch, and then back up through the groin and belly to the heart. The flow might circulate in the opposite direction, or simultaneously in both ways.

It can also help to track where sensation flows during sexual experiences, beyond what is happening in your genitals. Where else does arousal gather, and how does that sensation move around your body?

Partner energy circuits

Why is good sex so mind-blowing? At its core lies a sense of expansion of your own pleasure, connection with your lover's pleasure and being gripped by a nameless storm of love and lust that is beyond words or even full comprehension as it spreads far beyond the genitals. Your soft penis calls you out to notice the underlying arousal and energy storms that make sex so mind-blowing. Once your awareness is tuned in, you can turn up the amplifier dial.

Once you have noticed arousal sensations, energy flows and patterns in yourself, you can extend your awareness to include your partner. Here's one way of representing the pattern of loving energy exchange between partners, which draws on the wisdom of many yoga practices as well as Mantak Chia and others:

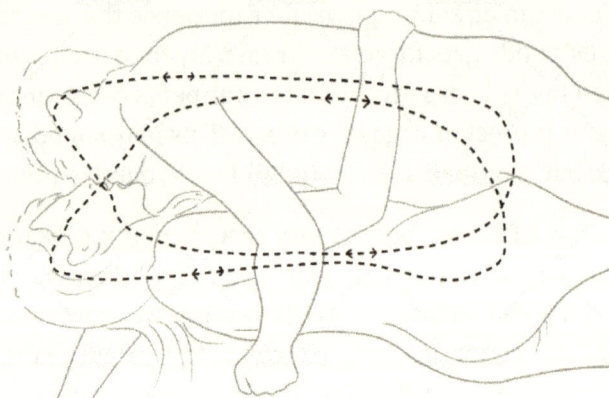

As the diagram suggests, both partners can practice opening your minds to sense the arousal flowing through your own bodies as you engage with each other.

Expanding your awareness like this can enable you to build arousal beyond erections, and regardless of the physical state of your penis. When both partners consciously and intentionally feed the energy flow, it is both sexually invigorating and one of the deepest acts of lovemaking possible.

To practice this sit or lie together, connecting sensually whatever way is comfortable. You might include some kind of genital-to-genital contact or simply be close and connected from head to toe. Sometimes cupping each other's genitals with your hands enhances awareness.

Maximising full-body skin to skin contact is most important. Then be still and breathe. Consciously project your love towards your partner.

Give it time.

Afterwards, you might share with each other what energy flows or circuits you became aware of.

4.3 Having hot sex with a soft penis

In many ways, humans in general are wired for climactic penetrative sex. It is the primary way our species reproduces. Particularly often, men feel driven to penetrate and thrust and thrill all the way to orgasm and ejaculation. It's probably the biggest sexual dilemma this book attempts to explore.

I get deeply satisfied by everything already described and explored in this book. Yet there are times when I just yearn for hot lustful sex. This was easy enough when I still had hard erections. I remember so many huge, thrusting, panting, bursting sexual peaks that left us, or me if solo, breathless, panting and completely drained of all that pent-up sexual heat.

Since I got soft, I still sometimes get conventional orgasms, but they usually take time and patience whether solo or partnered. I love all the soft touch and fluid, flowing connection, and sometimes I miss hot, hard, thrusting, lustful, explosive sex.

It's as if I need to let that kind of hot energy build up, sometimes for weeks, before the volcano is hot enough to burst. My partner seems to find something similar, without surgery and simply from the effects of age and hormonal changes.

Do you also experience this as a challenge? Research on men with erectile difficulties after prostate cancer treatment suggests that distress about orgasm is very common. For example, a 2002 study of 2,636 men on average four years after treatment at the Cleveland Clinic found that more men were distressed about orgasm problems than about erection problems.

This section draws together some opportunities to satisfy your hot-sex lust even though there is a soft penis in your life.

Partner witnessing self pleasuring

If you can still get really hot and orgasmic from self pleasuring, you might talk to your partner about either one or both of you doing it in each other's presence as described in Chapter 3.4. The sharing can make it even hotter than solo. If it works for you both, it can build intimacy - a bit like a shared secret. And if it helps you reach a hot climax with your partner, that is something to celebrate.

I struggle getting hard, I have struggled even before my tablets. My wife has helped a lot by changing how we have sex as my cock won't stay hard long enough for penetration. She will suck my cock and I normally have to finish off myself, which I enjoy having her watch. Then she will use my cock to orgasm herself by rubbing on me.
NB, aged 63, UK. On medication for enlarged prostate.

Find a version of penetration that works for you both

This might mean using a strap-on toy or supporting your soft penis with one of the medical or mechanical aids described in the previous chapter. Or perhaps your penis is just firm enough for the soft penetration described in Chapter 3.

Then let yourselves go wild. Amplify your arousal beyond erections. Make noise. Use your whole bodies. Try to find new ways to express your lust if your soft penis limits your thrusting movements. Partners might take over the thrusting role. Each let your partner know how much you enjoy making hot love.

Allow yourself to blow off steam alone ...

I've already suggested trying masturbation together with your partner. And it is okay to do it completely alone, including the practice of "edging" for extended periods of non-orgasmic arousal. And if you can reach a climax, allow yourself to flog that log until it bursts. Sometimes it takes so long that only its owner has the focus to continue. It's okay.

... and accept your limitations

Sometimes I find I just can't have the hot option – my spirit is willing but my body just stays limp and arousal dissipates. You might find this has happened to you too. It can feel awful, and it is what it is. It can help to measure your success in how quickly you get over the disappointment and live to try again another day and another way.

4.4 Evolving orgasms

Men with soft penises often struggle to have conventional orgasms the way they used to. The bad news is that this situation might be here for months, years or forever, and there is not usually any magic bullet to fix it.

The good news is that you can still have some kind of orgasm if you can expand your repertoire and be flexible in finding satisfaction. This is probably the most difficult and rewarding transformation of all. There are three broad areas to explore:

- Moving from genital to full body orgasms.
- Shifting the shape of orgasmic experience from short sharp peaks to longer slower climaxes, with the possibility of multiple orgasms.
- Expanding your definition of orgasm.

Full body orgasms

Most young men are convinced that ejaculation and orgasm are one and the same thing, because they usually occur together. The experience is usually ecstatic, strongly centred in the testicles and penis, includes pulsations so strong as to be jolting, and lasts a short time. This experience might be out of reach of your new body.

Erections, ejaculation and orgasm are all separate bodily functions and they are triggered by different parts of your neural network, as described simply and clearly in Cam Fraser's e-book **The New Male Sexuality**. As anybody who has had their prostate removed knows, you can still have intense orgasms without any form of ejaculation.

Orgasms can be stimulated by any and all of the ways using any or all of the body parts detailed in Chapter 3. Men can orgasm with or without erections. Orgasms can and do reverberate through the whole body. This is supported by a steady stream of clinical studies, going back at least as far as Rutgers University Professor Barry Komisaruk and American sexologist

Beverly Whipple's 2011 paper in the Journal of Sex and Relationship Therapy entitled *Non-genital orgasms.*

Some men report much more intense, full-bodied orgasms after prostate cancer treatment than before. I don't have hard data but I observe this to be true for me and I hear it is true for many others I trust. Post-prostatectomy orgasms can start at the toes and fingernails, and gather in the arms and legs, swirl around in groin and belly before fountaining out of penis regardless of hardness. Sometimes it feels as if they are breaking through the skull and connecting with the sun and sky and wind beyond.

Changing shape of orgasmic experience

The two most common changes for men moving from conventional erections and orgasms to sex beyond erections are:

- Sex with a soft penis takes much longer to ramp up and slow down.
- Several rolling climaxes can happen over an extended period, whereas hard penis sex is often dominated by a single intense peak followed by a longer refractory period.

The graphs below are not built on Masters and Johnson-style laboratory measurement. Rather they are sketches outlining the subjectively reported comparative experiences of men in my informal research group. Both graphs are to the same scales of overall sensation of arousal and time, with the horizontal dotted line representing the subjective arousal level of a man who feels "fully turned on."

Climax experience with hard erections

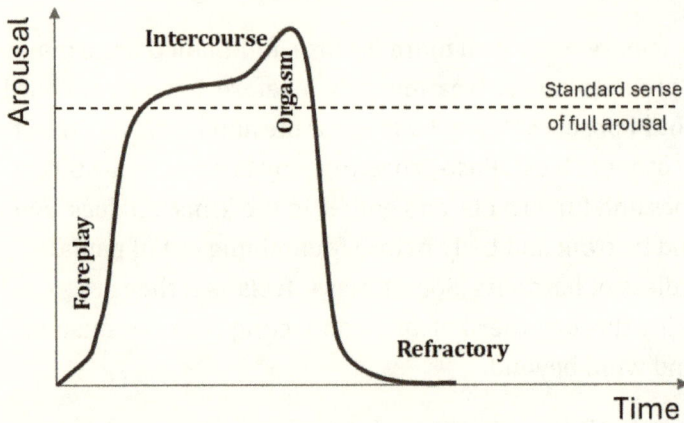

The first sketch shows the rapid ramping up of erection and arousal during what is often called foreplay, the hot sex of intercourse leading to an intense orgasm, followed quickly by the quick loss of erection and arousal known as a refractory period.

Climax experience with softer penis

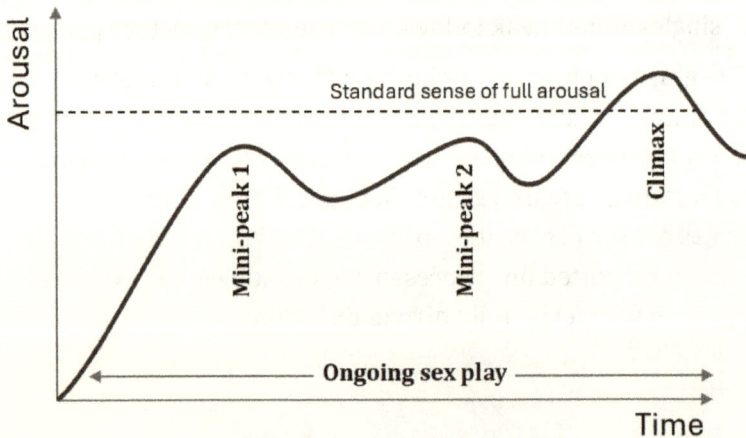

The second sketch represents a typical sexual experience for a man with a soft penis in which he seldom if ever reaches the same heights as in typical sex with a hard penis, but can experience multiple mini-peaks and little or no refractory period. It's been described as an extended rolling sense of ecstasy.

This opens the way for us to expand our definition of orgasm.

4.5 Redefining orgasm

Those with softer penises can struggle to reach strong, pulsating genital orgasms in the way they did when hard. What follows is for those who are experiencing soft penis pleasure but finding conventional orgasm elusive or out of reach.

I invite you to redefine orgasm for yourself to include all kinds of climax even if it doesn't include the same rhythmic pulsating jolts you used to experience. In polite circles, an orgasm is often referred to as a climax or a peak of passion. This points the way for us to become aware of and enjoy all our peaks of passion and climaxes as well as the sense of release that follows each peak.

Become expert at tracking arousal all over your body

Next time you get aroused, try to pay attention to all of the signals you get for that arousal – mental, physical, relational, maybe spiritual too. Set the goal of pleasure beyond erections: include but don't focus only on your genitals.

What is happening in your belly, your thighs, your ass? Feel the details of what is happening in your balls. What about your nipples, your chest, your arms and your neck? Feel how your internal temperature and pressure varies as you climb upwards in arousal.

Try to pay attention to the sensation of energy flows in your body and also energy exchanges with your partner, as described in the previous section on energy circuits.

Track every peak or climax

Be alert for rolling peaks and troughs in your combination of sexual arousal, energy flows and spiritual connectedness. If you let go of the drive for a conventional orgasm you can feel how your arousal climbs to its own peak before subsiding and recognise this as a form of orgasm. For me it includes something I can best describe as "clenching my brain" and then releasing it along with my erotic energy, my love, my pleasure.

This is also an orgasm, or at least a mini-peak.

Your soft penis can be your gateway into a much wider range of climactic sexual experience that goes far beyond erections.

Soft and hard

For most of those born into male bodies, hardness is wired into our lustful sexual selves. From before puberty, my penis got hard from certain kinds of touch and erotic imagination, and it just got harder and more enthusiastic about sex as time went on, until my prostate surgery. Now I'm softly sexual more than hard-driving.

Give yourself time to adjust to softer sexuality. You can learn from women – most women are wired to enjoy sex just as much as men, only with softer bodies. Many women have reported a wide variety of orgasmic or climax experiences. Several have contacted me after reading the first issue of this book and confirmed that their experiences parallel those described by men in this book.

4.6 Holistic satisfaction

You can maximise satisfaction by connecting sexually with the joys of your own body, as it is now. And if you have or want a partner, by connecting sexually with them with love and joy. Given the changes in your body, this will require:

- Erotic imagination and creativity.
- Adventurous exploration of pleasure, taking in all the capabilities of your body as it is now.
- Wisdom and skill in navigating energetic connection as well as new patterns of climax and satisfaction.
- An end to one-dimensional, genital-focused sex. Opening to new forms of sexual climax and satisfaction.

Many people will also find this a spiritual journey. While beyond the scope of this book, I believe that every time we suffer a significant loss, we are invited into spiritual awareness of our place in the world, the vastness of the universe, and the inevitability of birth, loss and death. Paradoxically, this can open us up to the choices that bring back love and joy in our lives.

4.7 Further exploration

It takes lots of practice to acclimate to long term changes in sexuality and satisfaction. You might find an activity in the list below that is helpful to you.

- Notice when your sexual play reaches a crescendo and then slackens without a conventional orgasm: practice celebrating the climax you just experienced. Enrol your partner's help. Slow down and feel the reverberations in your body, heart and mind. Recognise it for the climax, or peak of pleasure that it was.

- At first you might feel disappointed by mini-peaks without conventional orgasms. Give yourself time and track the ways you acclimatise to new and different arousal and satisfaction patterns.
- Track your sexual energy over a month or more. Record your sexual activity for that period. Identify patterns.
- Ask your partner what climaxes feel like to them, both your climaxes and theirs. Encourage them to describe how one climax might differ from another.
- Next time you just feel full of joy of life, while fully clothed, feel into the erotic nature of that joy.

Chapter 5 We are not alone

Wherever you are, however lonely you feel, you are truly not alone. This chapter is about reaching out to connect – informing yourself and those around you, and connecting with other human beings.

Most men and their partners benefit if they get support in adapting to erectile differences. There is no shame in seeking out the kind of help that really makes a difference in your unique situation. Here are some ideas to get you started.

5.1 Speak out about your experience

To create an environment where your erectile differences are taken for what they are – differences without shame – it is important that our different voices are heard in the world.

I respect and appreciate the work done by the annual Soft Cock Week in bringing us in from the cold and shaming place where we had been banished. My experience in the program has helped pave the way for me to write this book.

My desire for Soft Cock Week was to normalize a soft penis and expand our definition of "sex" so that a soft

> *penis didn't stop us from having sex. Bonus, I wanted*
> *to celebrate my love for softness.*
> Michelle Renee, founder of Soft Cock Week in 2022.

This initiative and others create more space in the world for every reader of this book to be who you are, as you are. You are welcome with whatever body parts you have and however they behave in sexual and other situations. Enjoy this freedom and build it outwards by telling others!

Probably the most important way to speak out about your experience is in your own circle of family and friends. However there is another option which might work for you too: you can write your story for others to read. In his book **The Wounded Storyteller,** Arthur Frank calls it "my attempt to widen the circle, to amplify and connect the voices that were telling tales about illness, so that all of us could feel less alone."

If this resonates with you, I encourage you to post your story on the platform of your choice. In drafting your story, one option is to use the "Share your Story" link on the Readers Portal for this book, which takes you to a template for sketching out your story. Anything you post on that form will be held strictly confidential until and unless you decide you want to make it public.

5.2 Inform yourself

The possibilities identified in this book are part of a bigger journey that goes well beyond what is covered here. And each reader's journey will be different. There are many relevant books, videos and articles for you to read along your journey. At the end of the book you will find some references and a brief selection of resources to support you. You can also access an

expanded version with clickable links in the Readers Portal at
www.beyonderections.com/readers.

5.3 Get help for your relationship

There is so much pain and shame attached to men with soft
penises. It is inevitable that your body changes will ask some
big changes of your relationship. Some couples find their way
through alone, but most couples need some help.

---

*My wife and I had some appointments with the
specialist psychosexual therapy nurse. We started by
talking about feelings before moving on to sensuality
and intimacy before we ever got round to mechanical
and chemical means of support.*

*[The nurse] told me that it was still possible to reach
orgasm without an erection but it would need a lot of
stimulation which would be enjoyable and we
therefore learned how to pleasure each other in
different ways that didn't involve penetrative sex but
did involve more use of sex toys as well as oral sex.*
Tony, 67, UK. Diagnosed with stage 4 cancer.

Many couples procrastinate about discussing the impact of
erectile differences on their relationship. It can feel awkward
and risky. If you need support in starting the conversation, you
might use this book as a conversation starter.

It can be very difficult to get into a constructive conversation
with your partner about such a touchy subject as sex,
particularly as your bodies have been or are changing. You
might really benefit from professional help, as Tony describes
above. Here are some options to consider.

5.4 Find people who can help you

As mentioned at the outset, your erection is a sensitive and holistic indicator of your health, and if it is behaving differently you should consult a doctor. If you are already under the care of a doctor or a team of doctors, don't wait for them to start a conversation about the sexual impact of your treatment. It is often up to you as the patient to tell your doctor you want a conversation about your sexual health in your next consultation, and to take your partner with you.

It is also good for your overall health if you find one or more non-medical people you trust, with whom you can talk as you grapple with sexual pleasure and intimacy in your changing body. Friends and lovers may be a good place to start, and they might not be enough.

You might benefit from a professional counsellor, therapist or coach and I encourage you to explore the options available to you.

Here are some categories of helping professionals you might search for and consult in your area:

- Family doctor
- Urologist and/or oncologist
- Pelvic floor specialist physical therapist/physiotherapist
- Sex educator or psychosocial sex educator
- Relationship coach or counsellor
- Sexologist
- Sexological bodyworker.

Some people are lucky enough to have access to integrated health care in their home neighbourhood, where you can get all or most of the above professional help through a single point of contact at your health service. Make the most of it if available.

In many parts of the world, you will need to create your own team by seeking out and consulting the range of helping professionals that can address the different dimensions of your challenges and changes.

5.5 *Supportive communities*

Responding to your erectile differences, the way they are affecting your sex life, your relationship and your way in the world as a man is so complex that you could probably benefit from a community of support. However, in the 21st century it is difficult to imagine your local neighbourhood community being able to overcome the taboos involved in talking openly about matters of sexual health.

The good news is that there are successful specialised communities growing up both online and in person. Here are a few suggestions to find one that suits you:

- Search online for local cancer and ED support groups. In your area, they might be organised by your health care authority, a religious institution or a prostate cancer foundation and possibly sponsored by international organisations like Movember.
- There is a selection of international online groups I can personally recommend in the Resources section and the Readers Portal.
- You can join the conversations supported by Soft Cock Week, www.softcockweek.com.

5.6 *Tracking progress*

Milestones and markers can be helpful to track progress on a long term project like yours. I suggest that you set up some kind of tracking for your journey across multiple dimensions using a device, a journal, or an app:

- Mindset – how are you thinking about yourself and your soft penis? You might track proportion of time in anger, sadness, adaptation and pleasure.
- Practical pleasure – I am talking about some appropriate form of notches in the bedpost. Remember to include solo pleasures and also different kinds of climaxes.
- Erectile function – including during conscious sexual situations, and spontaneous nocturnal erections, which are a good indicator of physical erectile health.
- Energetic adaptation – you could make notes or journal about the extent to which you are sexually satisfied.

There are some clever and comfortable wearable erection tracking devices that display data in a mobile app, such as those from Firmtech in the US and Adamhealth in the UK.

5.7 Further exploration

Here are some ideas to keep moving forward. I invite you to pick at least one to put into action.

- Talk to your partner about what kind of help might be good for your relationship. Start with "I think we need help coping with the changes." Identify at least one missing conversation and at least one change in the relationship that you both agree would help (even if you can't imagine how to achieve that outcome). Then contact a relationship coach or counsellor and ask them for help.
- Research some of the online resources mentioned in this book – you can use the Readers Portal from this book to get easy clickable links.
- Join a support group whether online or in person. You might need to try several to find the one that suits you.

- Start a sex journal tracking at least some aspect of your pleasure and sexual health.

Chapter 6 Action

Everything you have read, and all the practices you have tried out while reading this book, are designed to prepare you for ongoing action to save your own sex life. Please give yourself time, and keep reminding yourself that you are doing work for the whole world.

We are pioneering body positive, sex positive strategies that allow us to find joy where others might want to shame us. It takes courage and creativity and persistence.

It unavoidably takes time.

All this applies as much to your intimate partner or partners as to yourself. Partners are also bombarded with mainstream porn and shaming of erectile differences. The strength of your relationship can help them turn the corner too. You can support this by being candid with each other about your bodies and differing sexual energies, while avoiding judging each other's differences and changes.

I invite you to get into action – in mindset, in giving and receiving sexual pleasure, and in energetic awareness. You can both get help and be of help to others on this journey.

We are truly not alone.

You have a place as a person in the world. There are many ways to be powerful, sexy, loving and joyful beyond erections. Your loving kindness to yourself and those around you will expand those possibilities - not just for you but also for others.

I think it is time for men to claim vulnerability along with the power often assigned to us. It's also important to celebrate the qualities of adventurous exploration, drive and flexibility for all people, including those of us with soft penises.

Chapter 7 Resources

Everything that follows in this section is available online at the **Beyond Erections** Readers Portal, to give you easy access to clickable and updated links.

Visit the Readers Portal www.beyonderections.com/readers to get the latest on the resources listed below, as well as support for writing your own story of erectile difference and providing detailed feedback on this book.

The lists that follow include my personal suggestions based on experience. Feel free to search further online to suit your own preferences.

7.1 Free online resources

Where needed, hyperlinks are in the Readers Portal version of this list.

- www.ATouchySubject.com website founded and curated by psychologist and sexual health designer Victoria Cullen.
- Cam Fraser's downloadable e-book *The new male sexuality* and podcast *Men, Sex and Pleasure.*

- www.softcockweek.com website has a huge collection of resources. And look out for the next annual Soft Cock Week for a new wave of fresh thinking, actions and community building.
- *The Penis Project Podcast* co-founded by Melissa Hadley Barrett and Dr Jo Milios.

7.2 Online resources you might consider paying for

This short selection is limited to paid services I can personally recommend. Web links in the Readers Portal at BeyondErections.com/readers.

- Erotic massage "how to" guide videos including sensual *soft cock erotic massage* at EroticMassage.com.
- *Soft Penis Pleasure* masterclass by Tess Devèze.
- *Touchy Subject Hub* – penile rehabilitation community founded and curated by Victoria Cullen.

7.3 Sex aids

There is an unlimited array of toys, devices and other sex aids on the market. The Readers Portal includes links to the following selection of more personal stories and reviews to help you get started.

- Penis rings – I've reviewed of cheap and simple penis rings and the more sophisticated option that is now my favourite.
- Data logging – I've reviewed of wearable erection trackers.
- Strap on dildos – a user review from somebody I trust.
- Vacuum erection devices (penis pumps) – see Readers Portal for links to a variety of stories and experiences.

7.4 Support groups with free membership

I encourage you to find a group to join in your home area. If that doesn't work out, here are some that are accessible internationally. Web links in Readers Portal.

- *Gay, Bisexual Men and Transgender Women Prostate Cancer Support Group* on Facebook supported by US Prostate Cancer Foundation.
- *Intimacy and Cancer* – Facebook support group, mainly but not exclusively women dealing with the impact of cancer on sex and intimacy.
- *Prostate Cancer UK Community* – this is the best nationally-organised support group I have found.
- *Recovering Men* – live and very candid global conversations on Zoom.
- *Sex, Love and Prostate Cancer* – this is the most candid and open Facebook group I have found, and includes similar proportions of men and their partners.

7.5 Professional helpers

It's best to find the professional helper that suits you, if possible in your own area. Here are some individuals I can personally recommend:

- Delene van Dyk, RN, Sex educator, South Africa.
- Erica Leroye, Creative Body Release, USA.
- Melissa Hadley Barrett, nurse practitioner and sexologist focusing on erectile function, Australia.
- Michelle Renee, Human Connection Coach, USA.
- Tamboo Academy, and in particular their *Kadeisha: the art of conscious loving* series of in-depth workshops, South Africa.
- Victoria Cullen, founder of www.ATouchySubject.com, Australia.

7.6 More about quotes in the book

The people quoted in this book include many different races, gender identities and sexual orientations. This list identifies whether their stories are published, and if so I have included links in the Readers Portal.

- Catherine has written a series about her experiences recovering sexual pleasure with her husband after his prostate related surgery.
- Colleen has written a series about her experiences living with the author on his journey of prostate cancer and erectile differences.
- Johann has described his experience with a penile implant
- Gavin has described his prostate cancer and trans-Africa journey in depth.
- Pedro's blog includes a treasure trove for men dating with erectile differences.
- Pratap and his wife share practical details of their senior sex with erectile differences. Look out for their forthcoming book.
- Tony tells more about his life on hormone suppression treatment (ADT).

7.7 Bibliography

Books

Anand, M. *The Art of Sexual Ecstasy: The Path of Sacred Sexuality for Western Lovers* (1989)

Andrews, N. *The Book of Orgasms* (2000)

Chia, M. & Abrams, D. *The Multi-Orgasmic Man* (1996)

Chia, M., Abrams, D. & Abrams, R. C. *The Multi-Orgasmic Couple: Sexual Secrets Every Couple Should Know* (2000)

Dahl R. *Charlie and the Chocolate Factory* (1965)

Devèze, T. *A better normal: your guide to rediscovering intimacy after cancer* (2021)

Frank, A. *The Wounded Storyteller* (2nd edition, 2013)

Masters, W., Johnson, V., & Kolodny, R. *Heterosexuality* (1994)

Nagoski, E. *Come as You Are: The Surprising New Science that Will Transform Your Sex Life* (2015)

Nagoski, E. *Come Together: The Science (and Art!) of Creating Lasting Sexual Connections* (2024)

Perel, E. *Mating in Captivity: Unlocking Erotic Intelligence* (2007)

Research based articles

Bowie, J., Brunckhorst, O., Stewart, R., Dasgupta, P., & Ahmed, K. (2022). Body image, self-esteem, and sense of masculinity in patients with prostate cancer: a qualitative meta-synthesis. *Journal of cancer survivorship : research and practice*, *16*(1), 95–110. https://doi.org/10.1007/s11764-021-01007-9

Chambers, S. K., Chung, E., Wittert, G., & Hyde, M. K. (2017). Erectile dysfunction, masculinity, and psychosocial outcomes: a review of the experiences of men after prostate cancer treatment. *Translational andrology and urology*, *6*(1), 60–68. https://doi.org/10.21037/tau.2016.08.12

Daskivich, T. J., Naser-Tavakolian, A., Gale, R., Luu, M., Friedrich, N., Venkataramana, A., Khodyakov, D., Posadas, E., Sandler, H., Spiegel, B., & Freedland, S. J. (2024). Variation in communication of side effects in prostate cancer treatment consultations. *Prostate cancer and prostatic diseases*, *28*, 145-152. https://doi.org/10.1038/s41391-024-00806-2

Dowsett, G. W., Lyons, A., Duncan, D., & Wassersug, R. J. (2014). Flexibility in Men's Sexual Practices in Response to Iatrogenic Erectile Dysfunction after Prostate Cancer Treatment. *Sexual medicine, 2*(3), 115–120. https://doi.org/10.1002/sm2.32

Frey, A., Pedersen, C., Lindberg, H., Bisbjerg, R., Sønksen, J., & Fode, M. (2017). Prevalence and Predicting Factors for Commonly Neglected Sexual Side Effects to External-Beam Radiation Therapy for Prostate Cancer. *The journal of sexual medicine, 14*(4), 558–565. https://doi.org/10.1016/j.jsxm.2017.01.015

Frey, A., Sønksen, J., Jakobsen, H., & Fode, M. (2014). Prevalence and predicting factors for commonly neglected sexual side effects to radical prostatectomies: results from a cross-sectional questionnaire-based study. *The journal of sexual medicine, 11*(9), 2318–2326. https://doi.org/10.1111/jsm.12624

Fu, F., Duthie, C. J., Wibowo, E., Wassersug, R. J., & Walker, L. M. (2022). Openness to Using an External Penile Prosthesis for Maintaining Sexual Intimacy by Individuals with Erectile Dysfunction: A Cross-Sectional Study. *Sexual medicine, 10*(5), 100559. https://doi.org/10.1016/j.esxm.2022.100559

Hanna, P., Corre, C., Rapsey, C. & Wibowo, E. (2025). Description of how men achieve multiple orgasms, *Sexual and Relationship Therapy.* https://doi.org/10.1080/14681994.2025.2451995

Kessler, A., Sollie, S., Challacombe, B., Briggs, K., & Van Hemelrijck, M. (2019). The global prevalence of erectile dysfunction: a review. *BJU international, 124*(4), 587–599. https://doi.org/10.1111/bju.14813

Kinnaird, W., Schartau, P., Kirby, M., Jenkins, V., Allen, S., Payne, H. (2025). Sexual Dysfunction in Prostate Cancer Patients According to Disease Stage and Treatment Modality. *Journal of Clinical Oncology*, Volume 41, 2025, 103801.
DOI: 10.1016/j.clon.2025.103801

Komisaruk, B. R., & Whipple, B. (2011). Non-genital orgasms. *Sexual and Relationship Therapy*, *26*(4), 356–372.
https://doi.org/10.1080/14681994.2011.649252

Ladegaard, P. B. J., Mortensen, J., Skov-Jeppesen, S. M., & Lund, L. (2021). Erectile Dysfunction A Prospective Randomized Placebo-Controlled Study Evaluating the Effect of Low-Intensity Extracorporeal Shockwave Therapy (LI-ESWT) in Men With Erectile Dysfunction Following Radical Prostatectomy. *Sexual medicine*, *9*(3), 100338.
https://doi.org/10.1016/j.esxm.2021.100338

Lyons, K. S., Winters-Stone, K. M., Bennett, J. A., & Beer, T. M. (2016). The effects of partnered exercise on physical intimacy in couples coping with prostate cancer. *Health psychology: official journal of the Division of Health Psychology, American Psychological Association*, *35*(5), 509–513.
https://doi.org/10.1037/hea0000287

McKinlay J. B. (2000). The worldwide prevalence and epidemiology of erectile dysfunction. *International journal of impotence research*, *12 Suppl 4*, S6–S11.
https://doi.org/10.1038/sj.ijir.3900567

Meissner, V. H., Dumler, S., Kron, M., Schiele, S., Goethe, V. E., Bannowsky, A., Gschwend, J. E., & Herkommer, K. (2020). Association between masturbation and functional outcome in the postoperative course after nerve-sparing radical prostatectomy. *Translational andrology and urology*, *9*(3), 1286–1295.
https://doi.org/10.21037/tau.2020.03.19

Ralph S. (2021). Developing UK Guidance on How Long Men Should Abstain from Receiving Anal Sex before, During and after Interventions for Prostate Cancer. *Clinical oncology (Royal College of Radiologists (Great Britain))*, *33*(12), 807–810. https://doi.org/10.1016/j.clon.2021.07.010

Rawla P. (2019). Epidemiology of Prostate Cancer. *World journal of oncology*, *10*(2), 63–89. https://doi.org/10.14740/wjon1191

Schover, L.R., Fouladi, R.T., Warneke, C.L., Neesec L., Klein, E.A., Zippe, C., Kupelian, P.A., Defining sexual outcomes after treatment for localized prostate carcinoma. *Cancer.* 2002 Oct 15;95(8):1773–1785. DOI: 10.1002/cncr.10848

Schwartz, A. N., Wang, K. Y., Mack, L. A., Lowe, M., Berger, R. E., Cyr, D. R., & Feldman, M. (1989). Evaluation of normal erectile function with color flow Doppler sonography. *AJR. American journal of roentgenology*, *153*(6), 1155–1160. https://doi.org/10.2214/ajr.153.6.1155

Tsang, V. W. L., Skead, C., Wassersug, R. J., & Palmer-Hague, J. L. (2019). Impact of prostate cancer treatments on men's understanding of their masculinity. *Psychology of Men & Masculinities, 20*(2), 214–225. https://doi.org/10.1037/men0000184

Tutolo, M., Briganti, A., Suardi, N., Gallina, A., Abdollah, F., Capitanio, U., Bianchi, M., Passoni, N., Nini, A., Fossati, N., Rigatti, P., & Montorsi, F. (2012). Optimizing postoperative sexual function after radical prostatectomy. *Therapeutic advances in urology*, *4*(6), 347–365. https://doi.org/10.1177/1756287212450063

Ussher, J. M., Perz, J., Rose, D., Dowsett, G. W., Chambers, S., Williams, S., Davis, I., & Latini, D. (2017). Threat of Sexual

Disqualification: The Consequences of Erectile Dysfunction and Other Sexual Changes for Gay and Bisexual Men With Prostate Cancer. *Archives of sexual behavior, 46*(7), 2043–2057. https://doi.org/10.1007/s10508-016-0728-0

Usta, M.F., Gabrielson, A.T. & Bivalacqua, T.J. Low-intensity extracorporeal shockwave therapy in the treatment of erectile dysfunction following radical prostatectomy: a critical review. (2019). *Int J Impot Res* **31**, 231–238. https://doi.org/10.1038/s41443-019-0121-3

Walker, L. M., & Robinson, J. W. (2012). Sexual adjustment to androgen deprivation therapy: struggles and strategies. *Qualitative health research, 22*(4), 452–465. https://doi.org/10.1177/1049732311422706

Wassersug R. J. (2016). Maintaining intimacy for prostate cancer patients on androgen deprivation therapy. *Current opinion in supportive and palliative care, 10*(1), 55–65. https://doi.org/10.1097/SPC.0000000000000190

Wassersug, R. J. (2014). Prostate cancer, gonadal hormones, and my brain. *Journal of sex & marital therapy, 40*(5), 355–357. https://doi.org/10.1080/0092623X.2014.921477

Wassersug, R., & Wibowo, E. (2017). Non-pharmacological and non-surgical strategies to promote sexual recovery for men with erectile dysfunction. *Translational andrology and urology, 6*(Suppl 5), S776–S794. https://doi.org/10.21037/tau.2017.04.09

Wibowo, E., & Wassersug, R. J. (2016). Multiple Orgasms in Men—What We Know So Far. *Sexual Medicine Reviews.* 4(2), 136-148. https://doi.org/10.1016/j.sxmr.2015.12.004

Wittmann, D., Foley, S., & Balon, R. (2011). A biopsychosocial approach to sexual recovery after prostate cancer surgery: the role of grief and mourning. *Journal of sex & marital therapy*, *37*(2), 130–144. https://doi.org/10.1080/0092623X.2011.560538

Yates, P., Carter, R., Peniserell, R., Cowan, D., Dixon, C., Magnus, A., Newton, R. U., Hart, N. H., Galvão, D. A., Baguley, B., Denniston, N., Skinner, T., Couper, J., Emery, J., Frydenberg, M., & Liu, W. H. (2021). An integrated multicomponent care model for men affected by prostate cancer: A feasibility study of TrueNTH Australia. *Psycho-oncology*, *30*(9), 1544–1554. https://doi.org/10.1002/pon.5729

Other articles

Cooper, S. *Taboos in Treating Men's Sexual, Erectile, and Mental Health.* Psychology Today. Nov 19, 2024.

Fisher, J. *5 stages of grief: Coping with the loss of a loved one.* Harvard Health Publishing, Harvard Medical School. Dec 12, 2023.

Goldstein, I. *The Central Mechanisms of Sexual Function.* Boston University Medical Centre. 2021.

Kenny, S. *In Chicago, a New Approach to Gay and Bisexual Men With Prostate Cancer.* New York Times. Dec 7, 2021.

Kramer, J. The Body Electric School. 1984. https://bodyelectric.org/about-us/our-history/

Lanquist, L and Borges, A. *How to prepare for anal sex, according to actual doctors.* Self.com. 2020.

Middelmann, M. *Let's Talk About Erectile Dysfunction: How my prostate cancer experience is helping make ED more discussable for me.* Psychology Today, May 3, 2021

Middelmann, M. *Assumptions and Taboos: Breaking down barriers to men's sexual health and relationships.* Institute of Psychosexual Medicine Journal, 83, 10-15. 2024.

Sexual Medicine Society of North America, *What Is Sensate Focus and How Does It Work?*

Acknowledgements

Many people have contributed to the creation of this book. I am grateful to you all, whether or not you are named here. You have made this a better book. I remain responsible for the final outcome including any limitations or mistakes that emerge.

The extraordinary global community brought together around my website at www.recoveringman.net has been a central inspiration for this book. Many have allowed me to publish their intimate stories on the blog. Some have shared very deeply in the global Recovering Man support group – because of the confidential nature of the group I neither quote from its contents nor mention participants' names.

This whole journey wouldn't have happened without the enthusiastic support of Colleen Dawson. She has brought her vast professional experience as an editor and publisher to this project. I treasure our ongoing life and love partnership which is now well into its fifth decade.

Erica Leroye and Michael Scott both read and commented incisively and very helpfully on my manuscript on an unreasonably tight schedule.

Vanissar Tarakali opened my mind to the possibility of writing a book that combines memoir, informal research and original content. Michelle Renee expanded public conversation about erectile differences by initiating Soft Penis Week in 2022, and Erica Leroye has carried that baton further since 2024.

Generous couples including Pratap and Jeannie, Michael and Ann, Tom and Lorraine, Rhys and Linda, Jim and Crystal, Catherine and her husband, and many more have shared their experiences in ways that open my mind and my heart. Many of their stories are published on the Recovering Man website.

Dr Jo Milios, Hester van Aswegen, Pierre Röscher and Daniel Devere have helped me tremendously with pelvic floor physiotherapy. Richard Wassersug's sexology research inspired me, and he also reviewed an early version of my manuscript.

Victoria Cullen was the first person in the world I found who provided down to earth and detailed help in grappling with my new body. Melissa Hadley Barrett and Cam Fraser pushed me over the edge into my first open public sharing of the impact of erectile differences on my life and relationships by interviewing me on their podcasts in 2021.

Jim Mitchell, James McCleary, Eugene Oppelt, Paul Abro and the men of the Mankind Project all around the world were some of the first to teach me how to be open, vulnerable, brave and kind with other men.

The heritage that informs Chapter 3 includes the *Sensate Focus* approach pioneered by Masters and Johnson, which has been adapted and advanced by Joe Kramer and the sexological bodywork methodologies he helped set up.

My family has supported and delighted me through life and through prostate cancer. And they have found good ways to be with my ongoing and outspoken interest in sex.

I am grateful to all these people as well as those who remain anonymous for your help, support, love and inspiration.

About the author

Until 2020, Mish circled the globe, consulting and coaching in large organisations grappling with complex change in Africa, Asia, Europe and North America. Before he became a coach in 2007, he co-founded and was first CEO of a successful software and services company in Johannesburg, South Africa. Prior to that he taught A level Physics in Harare, Zimbabwe in the 1980s. He was born in Cape Town as a privileged white man under the apartheid system.

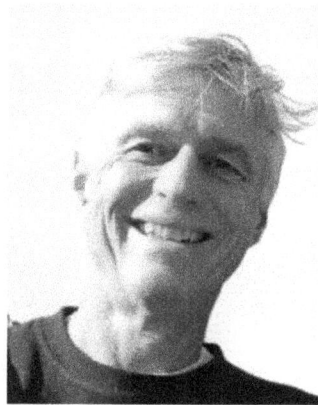

Since his radical prostatectomy because of prostate cancer in February 2020, Mish has continued working worldwide as a coach, consultant and trainer of organisational and relationship coaches, but on a more modest schedule. Soon after the operation, Mish began blogging his experiences on RecoveringMan.net and drew in others to tell their stories. He set up and has facilitated monthly international online support groups since 2020 with men around the world who have been diagnosed with prostate cancer or experience difficulties with their sexual health.

The tens of thousands of visitors to his website and hundreds who have participated in the discussions revealed overwhelming interest in how to have a satisfying sex life beyond erections – and that this desire is not confined to those who have had prostate cancer.

His explorations have led to his participation in a variety of public conversations and podcasts, including *The Penis Project*, Cam Fraser's *Men, Sex & Pleasure*, *La Nogalera* (Spanish), CRR Global's *Relationship Matters*, and *Soft Cock Week*. Mish was given the Ron Hering Mission of Service Award in 2021, awarded to men involved in the Mankind Project who excel in missions of service to the wider community, for his work on the Recovering Man support groups and website. In 2023 Mish delivered a paper to the Annual Clinical Meeting of the UK Institute for Psychosexual Medicine.

He and his life partner Colleen have two adult sons, whom they followed to North America in 2023. Mish and Colleen now live near the shore of Lake Ontario in Toronto, Canada.

www.ingramcontent.com/pod-product-compliance
Lightning Source LLC
Chambersburg PA
CBHW022340280326
41934CB00006B/708